Quick Reference
to
WOUND CARE

Palliative, Home, and Clinical Practices

FOURTH EDITION

Edited by
Pamela Brown, RN, BSN, MEd, CWON
Certified Wound and Ostomy Nurse
St. Joseph-Baptist Hospital
Tampa, Florida

JONES & BARTLETT
LEARNING

World Headquarters
Jones & Bartlett Learning
5 Wall Street
Burlington, MA 01803
978-443-5000
info@jblearning.com
www.jblearning.com

Jones & Bartlett Learning books and products are available through most bookstores and online booksellers. To contact Jones & Bartlett Learning directly, call 800-832-0034, fax 978-443-8000, or visit our website, www.jblearning.com.

The authors, editor, and publisher have made every effort to provide accurate information. However, they are not responsible for errors, omissions, or for any outcomes related to the use of the contents of this book and take no responsibility for the use of the products and procedures described. Treatments and side effects described in this book may not be applicable to all people; likewise, some people may require a dose or experience a side effect that is not described herein. Drugs and medical devices are discussed that may have limited availability controlled by the Food and Drug Administration (FDA) for use only in a research study or clinical trial. Research, clinical practice, and government regulations often change the accepted standard in this field. When consideration is being given to use of any drug in the clinical setting, the health care provider or reader is responsible for determining FDA status of the drug, reading the package insert, and reviewing prescribing information for the most up-to-date recommendations on dose, precautions, and contraindications, and determining the appropriate usage for the product. This is especially important in the case of drugs that are new or seldom used.

Production Credits
Publisher: Kevin Sullivan
Acquisitions Editor: Amanda Harvey
Editorial Assistant: Sara Bempkins
Associate Production Editor: Sara Fowles
Associate Marketing Manager: Katie Hennessy
V.P., Manufacturing and Inventory Control: Therese Connell
Composition: Circle Graphics
Cover Design: Kristin E. Parker
Cover Image: © Comstock/Thinkstock
Printing and Binding: Malloy, Inc.
Cover Printing: Malloy, Inc.

Some images in this book feature models. These models do not necessarily endorse, represent, or participate in the activities represented in the images.

Library of Congress Cataloging-in-Publication Data
Quick reference to wound care : palliative, home, and clinical practices/[edited by] Pamela Brown. — 4th ed.
    p. ; cm.
  Includes bibliographical references and index.
  ISBN 978-1-4496-0011-2 (pbk.)
  I. Brown, Pamela A.
  [DNLM: 1. Skin Ulcer—nursing—Handbooks. 2. Wounds and Injuries—nursing—Handbooks. 3. Nursing Records—Handbooks. 4. Wound Healing—Handbooks. WR 39]
  617.1'06—dc23
                                                                                          2011043986

6048

Printed in the United States of America
16 15 14 13 12   10 9 8 7 6 5 4 3 2 1

DEDICATION

This fourth edition is dedicated to the doctors and nurses at Mission Hospital in Asheville, NC who worked tirelessly to save my son from death in 2010, and in the process to heal his wounds.

CONTENTS

PART II—BASICS OF WOUND MANAGEMENT

PART III—WOUND TYPES COMMONLY SEEN BY HEALTHCARE PROFESSIONALS

PART IV—SPECIFIC APPLICATIONS OF
WOUND CARE PRACTICE

ACKNOWLEDGMENTS

A special thank you to my husband, Warren Clark, for his assistance in editing and composing this book. I also want to thank nurses and caregivers who work hard to provide compassionate healing care. This book is for them.

I want to thank the contributing writers who bring their knowledge from many different health-care arenas where wound care is practiced. I am grateful for Donna Oddo, who wrote Chapters 5, 6, and 11. I also appreciate Jo Patterson's willingness to share her passion that healthcare professionals have access to the most current information available to care for persons with wounds. Julie Maloy has been a major contributor to this book. Dilicia Marzorati, Registered Clinical Dietician at St. Joseph's Hospital in Tampa, Florida, provided current information and guidance on nutrition and wound healing. Special thank you to MariJo Letizia who wrote a new chapter on palliative wound care, and to Karen Lou Kennedy-Evans, S. Kwon Lee, and Shirley Grant who co-authored a new chapter on long-term care. And, finally, thanks to Ben Peirce, who made major updates to the chapter on home health wound documentation.

—*Pamela Brown*

CONTRIBUTORS

Pamela Brown, RN, BSN, MEd, CWON

Certified Wound and Ostomy Nurse
St. Joseph-Baptist Hospital
Tampa, Florida

Shirley Grant, LPN

Administrative and Research Assistant
TLC HealthCare, Corp.
Tucson, Arizona

Karen Lou Kennedy-Evans, RN, FNP, APRN-BC

LLC Wound and Skin Management
Tucson, Arizona

S. Kwon Lee, MD, FACS, CWSP, FACCWS

Chief Medical Officer
Northeast Surgical Wound Care, Inc.
Chardon, Ohio

MariJo Letizia, PhD, RN, APN/ANP-BC

Professor and Associate Dean of MSN/DNP Programs
Loyola University
Chicago, Illinois

Julie Phelps Maloy, ARNP, MS, CWOCN

Program Co-Director
WICKS Educational Associates, Inc.
Mechanicsburg, Pennsylvania

Christopher A. Morrison, MD, CSW

Medical Director & President
Nautilus Health Care Group
Tierra Verde, Florida

Donna Oddo, RN, BSN, CWOCN

Customer Support Convatec
New Port Richey, Florida

Jo A. Patterson, CHRN, CWS, DAPWCA

Clinical Nurse
Postanesthesia Care Unit
Wilford Hall Ambulatory Surgical Unit
Lackland AFB, Texas

Ben Peirce, RN, CWOCN

Asst. VP for Clinical Practice
Gentiva Health Services
Melville, New York

INTRODUCTION

The authors of the first three editions are pleased that this book has been so well received. Here's what's new with this fourth edition:

A chapter on palliative wound care addresses the special needs of patients, often near the end of life with nonhealing wounds. Treatment goals are to stabilize the wound, prevent new wounds, and manage symptoms, such as pain, with a focus on the quality of the patient's life.

The chapter on long-term care has been redone by new contributors, Karen Lou Kennedy-Evans, Shirley Grant, and Dr. Kwon Lee, who are widely respected experts on wound care. This chapter walks the reader through the recent federal changes in documentation and assessment of patients with wounds in long-term care facilities and covers a wide range of treatment options.

The home care chapter is written by one of the top home care experts in the United States in the area of wound care. This redone chapter covers several significant Centers for Medicare and Medicaid Services (CMS) changes since the third edition was published.

The first chapter now has a section written by a physician on how to communicate about wound care between doctors and nurses.

Chapter by chapter, the book has been updated to reflect current wound care treatments and products. Scientifically based wound care is recognized as a key factor in helping patients heal more quickly. Changes in Medicare and managed care are demanding more cost-effective plans of treatment. A huge industry has built up around the heightened interest in wound care.

Even with major advances in wound care in the last 30 years, wound management in many settings may not be scientifically based. For optimal healing to occur, a plan must be developed that will incorporate wound etiology, appropriate assessment skills, principles of wound healing, scientifically based treatments, and prevention measures. The plan needs to include appropriate goals for wound healing and reevaluation of the process at regular intervals.

The main purpose of this book is to provide healthcare professionals with information that is easy to use, so they can provide optimal wound care in the most cost-effective manner. **This is a nuts-and-bolts book** that covers the basics in wound care from A to Z. The most common wound types are illustrated with color photographs. There are numerous exhibits to aid clinicians in assessment, documentation, and day-to-day treatment of wounds.

Part I includes a chapter written by a physician. This chapter gives a concise description of what a physician needs to know when developing a plan of care for a patient with a wound. This section also includes a chapter with step-by-step instructions for accurate assessment and documentation of wounds. Accurate assessment and documentation are important for communication between medical professionals and directly affect reimbursement issues.

Part II addresses the normal healing process, basics of wound management and topical treatments. Using the information in these chapters, a clinician can assess the patient, develop an individualized care plan, determine the appropriate healing goals and match the dressing to the wound.

Part III includes a new chapter on palliative wound care. Other chapters focus on specific wound types commonly seen by healthcare professionals. The etiology of the wound types, treatments, and prevention are included. Teaching guides, case studies, and tips from experience punctuate the main points covered in this section

Part IV has major updates on issues specific to home health care and extended care facilities. Criteria for admission, reimbursement issues, and documentation are discussed for each setting.

Contributors to this book include certified wound and ostomy nurses with extensive experience in home, hospital and extended care settings; physicians who specialize in wound care; and an assistant vice president for clinical practice and wound care for a national home health agency. For more in-depth information on topics covered in this book, or for wound types not addressed, the reader should refer to more comprehensive wound care resources. This book is designed to be a quick reference.

Assessment and Documentation

Initial Wound Assessment and Communication

Christopher A. Morrison
S. Kwon Lee

Thanks to advancements in technology, our ability to communicate with one another is unprecedented. However, it seems that communication among health-care providers regarding patient care is at an all-time low. Health care is trying to cope with increased patient volumes, decreased revenue, and the burden of documentation. As medicine continues to subspecialize, providers must communicate with greater precision. This is certainly true for wound care. Very often the prescribing physician relies on communication with the treating nurse to help determine an appropriate wound care treatment plan.

Communication needs to cover the diagnosis and treatment of the physical and mental characteristics of a patient. This combination of physical and mental assessment is especially important for those with nonhealing wounds. Popular belief holds that advanced technologies have improved our healing outcomes. Actually, the strongest gains in wound healing have come from sharpened assessment and aggressive treatment of the underlying factors that can impede healing. That means a thorough assessment is a must when a patient is admitted to your agency or facility. As the treating nurse, your job is to take an accurate history and to examine the patient. Then you need to describe your findings, document them in the medical record, and communicate your findings with the treating physician. All the nurses caring for the patient need to follow through by assessing wound progress accurately and communicating effectively with the rest of the treating team. This is important not only for the care of the patient but also because of today's medical malpractice climate.

COMMUNICATIONS WITH PHYSICIANS: TAKING THE NEXT STEP

S. Kwon Lee

I am in full agreement with Dr. Morrison when he says that communication holds the key to improving wound outcomes. However, there is still a real communication gap on what to do with the information, especially among physicians.

Old traditional and unproven methods still remain the "standard of care" in many areas of this country. So communicating the information will take you only halfway down the road to success. There must be better understanding of what to do with the information and a common language established when it comes to advanced wound care if we are going to achieve better outcomes.

A simple checklist of things to do in helping to get physician buy-in and understanding will go a long way toward reaching common ground and a consistent approach to wound management.

1. Understand and adopt moist wound healing protocol. "Gauze has no cause." Gauze is not moist wound healing. Physicians must be taught the concept of moist wound healing.
2. Standardize wound product choices. One of the things that frustrates physicians and nurses is that "there are 2,500 products, so which ones do I choose?" Standardize your approach by looking at products by **category** rather than by **brand name**. Learn 8 to 10 different types of product categories and then utilize them on a regular basis. In addition, if you choose from just one or two product lines, there will be less confusion about products. Inservice training about products is vital. It is much easier if you commit to use one or two companies, who will then provide the educational support.
3. Convince the physicians. Educate physicians to adopt modern wound care, but realize it may not be easy. Develop just one or two physicians as wound care champions. Get them to incorporate modern wound care as part of their practice. Let them help educate and convince other physicians. Physicians must understand that "wet to dry" is a mechanical debridement technique and not a healing technique.
4. Develop case examples. Physicians need to see the outstanding results that can be achieved with the variety of newer dressings and devices. Put together cases to show physicians that their patient will heal their wound faster with less pain and bleeding. Seeing is believing. This is true for wound care as well.

So, communicate the important and vital information. Then take the next step to help physicians and other clinicians learn that there is such a thing as advanced wound care. Demonstrate through case studies that it has true benefit to patients and clinicians alike.

MEDICAL HISTORY

The patient's medical history is key to understanding possible physiological influences on wound healing. This information can help identify local and systemic risk factors that impede wound healing. Some of these include:

- tissue oxygen perfusion
- edema

- bacterial bioburden
- pressure, shear, friction
- nutritional status
- central circulatory dysfunction including congestive heart failure and chronic obstructive pulmonary disease
- chronic illness including diabetes mellitus, renal insufficiency, and malignancy
- dermatological abnormalities including skin cancer, dermatitis, previous radiation, and scarring
- inflammatory or autoimmune disorders including vasculitis, rheumatoid arthritis, scleroderma, and lupus
- coagulation disorders
- immunosuppression including corticosteroids and chemotherapy
- age
- physiologic and psychological stress

WOUND HISTORY

The patient's wound healing history can yield helpful information for implementing the wound care plan:

- Does the patient have a history of previous nonhealing wounds?
- How long has the patient had the current wound?
- What caused or may have caused the current wound?
- Were there past treatments used on the wound? Were they successful?
- Who was the treating physician?
- Was any diagnostic testing undertaken (noninvasive vascular studies, radiographs, other imaging studies, or cultures)?

Wound Assessment

Accurate assessment of the wound is crucial for determining appropriate topical and systemic therapies that might aid in healing.

- Record length, width, and depth of the wound.
- Note depth and location of any undermining or tunneling. Use the face of a clock for orientation with 12 o'clock being toward the head of the patient and 6 o'clock toward the feet. Undermining is defined as space that extends under the skin or superficial tissue and usually involves a larger area of the border of the wound (i.e., 1.5 cm undermining from 3 o'clock to 7 o'clock). A tunnel is a narrow passageway extending from the open wound under intact tissue (i.e., tunneling 3 cm at 5 o'clock). A tunnel has an end and is dead space. Do not confuse a tunnel with a fistula. A fistula is an abnormal

passage connecting two or more structures or spaces. It can connect one body cavity or hollow organ to another or to the skin.

- Describe the condition of the wound tissue. Mention the presence, color, and percentage of healthy granulation tissue, fibrous tissue or slough, necrotic tissue, eschar, or gangrene.
- Report any exposed tendon, ligament, muscle, or bone, as well as its color and overall appearance.
- Describe the characteristics of the wound drainage. Note the amount (large, moderate, minimal) and type of fluid (serous, serosanguineous, bloody, purulent).
- Inspect the condition of the periwound area, noting erythema, warmth, maceration, fluctuance, scarring, and dermatitis.
- If the wound involves a lower extremity, a thorough physical examination can give immediate insight into the underlying etiologies of nonhealing. Note skin color and quality (normal, thin, shiny, dry, scaly, erythematous, brawny, etc.). Note presence of edema (1+ to 4+) and any weeping or drainage from the leg. Record the temperature of the legs, feet, and toes (warm, cool, cold). Note the presence or absence of hair on the legs, feet, and toes. Check for capillary refill at the toenail beds (i.e., less than 3 seconds). Assess the femoral, popliteal, dorsalis pedis, and posterior tibial arteries.
- Because pain is now considered the fifth vital sign, ask the patient to assess the pain on a scale of 1 to 10. Pain provides important information and can have a significant impact on the patient's quality of life and ability to heal. An extremely painful wound can signify an inflammatory condition (pyoderma gangrenosum, vasculitis) or infection. Ischemic ulcers can also be very painful and may indicate the presence of underlying peripheral vascular disease. As pain is usually subjective, it is best to have the patient rate his or her pain on a scale of 1 to 10 (10 being the worst pain they have ever felt).

Risk Factors

To be as successful as possible in healing chronic wounds, you must be proactive. You must assess the patient as a whole, including underlying risk factors that may play a part in nonhealing. This comprehensive assessment aids healing outcomes and can help prevent further problems.

- Flexion contractures of the extremities that place excessive axial loading force on the wound or other bony prominence should be identified. To decrease the likelihood of poor outcomes, the recommendation of appropriate off-loading devices is important.
- Note the type of mattress, cushion, and any other off-loading pressure devices that the patient is using. Also, communicate where (and in which position) the patient spends his or her time.

- A nutritional assessment, if available, should be communicated.
- Note any known history of noncompliance or inability to follow instructions.

The wound assessment report to the attending physician should be a concise 2- to 3-minute summary. It should contain wound characteristics and descriptions and all other pertinent patient information. With this type of initial wound assessment and communication, the patient will benefit from a team healthcare approach. Appropriate initial treatment increases likelihood for a positive outcome. **Exhibit 1–1** is a sample wound report prepared for a physician. **Exhibit 1–2** is a blank copy of the report.

Exhibit 1–1 Sample Wound Report

WOUND REPORT SHEET

Medical Record #:_____

Date: _____ Patient Name: _____ Date of Birth: _____

Diagnoses: __UTI, IDDM, CHF_____

Wound Location: __Stage III Pressure Ulcer in the coccygeal area_____
(Use additional page for additional wounds)

Pressure Ulcer: Stage ___III_____; or Partial Thickness _____ Full Thickness _____

Size: _3.5cm_ L × _5.3cm_ W × _2.0cm_ D; undermining/tunneling _____ cms. located @ _____ o'clock

Wound Bed: _45__ % Red, _55__ % Yellow, _____ % Black, _____ Other (Describe)_____

Wound Margins: __Macerated and Open_____ (Closed, reddened, warm, tender, macerated, denuded)

Exudate Amount: __Dressing saturated at change_____ Type: __serous____, Odor noted (Y/N): __No_____

Pain Assessment: __Medicated for dressing change; pain level 6 prior to medication_____

Current Treatment: __Wet to dry dressing changes BID_____

Impressions: __Wet to dry dressing changes are painful. Periwound is macerated from excessive moisture.__
Increase of approx. 10% amt. of healthy red tissue within the last week. Yellow tissue has decreased.
_____

Recommendations: __Stop wet to dry BID changes. Begin wound care daily with calcium alginate to control__
the exudate, decrease maceration. Apply cover dressing._____
_____

Name of person making report (Please Print): __Jane Doe RN_____

Signature of person making report: __Jane Doe RN_____ Phone Number: __818-888-8888_____

Physician: Please write your orders for wound care below, and contact _____HH Supervisor_____ **at**
Phone: _____ **Fax:** _____
Physician: Please print & sign your name below:

Doctor's Name: _____ **Signature:** _____

Exhibit 1–2 Sample Wound Report

WOUND REPORT SHEET   Medical Record #:_____

Date: _____ Patient Name: _____ Date of Birth: _____

Diagnoses: _____

Wound Location: _____
(Use additional page for additional wounds)

Pressure Ulcer: Stage _____; or Partial Thickness _____ Full Thickness _____

Size: _____ L × _____ W × _____ D; undermining/tunneling _____ cms. located @ _____ o'clock

Wound Bed: _____ % Red, _____ % Yellow, _____ % Black, _____ Other (Describe)_____

Wound Margins: _____ (Closed, reddened, warm, tender, macerated, denuded)

Exudate Amount: _____ Type: _____, Odor noted (Y/N): _____

Pain Assessment: _____

Current Treatment: _____

Impressions: _____
_____
_____

Recommendations: _____
_____
_____

Name of person making report (Please Print): _____

Signature of person making report: _____ Phone Number: _____

Physician: Please write your orders for wound care below, and contact _____ **at**
Phone: _____ **Fax:** _____
Physician: Please print & sign your name below:

Doctor's Name: _____ **Signature:** _____

Assessment and Documentation for Wounds: A Step-by-Step Process

Pamela Brown

Wound care begins with a careful and thorough assessment. The clinician should determine the etiology of the wound and any factors that could affect the healing process. Ongoing assessment should be done at regular intervals, ideally weekly, to determine healing progress. Consistency in wound assessment is important. The wound should be evaluated with the patient in the same position each time and preferably by the same clinician. Photography or tracings can be used as documentation tools and can provide helpful information. Accurate documentation enables critical evaluation of the wound healing progress. It can also directly affect reimbursement and help protect clinicians against litigation.

WOUND CLASSIFICATION

Skin, the body's largest organ, is divided into two layers: the epidermis and the dermis. Underneath these lie subcutaneous tissue, fascia, muscle, and bone. The classification of a wound is determined by the number of layers it penetrates.

1. Partial-thickness wounds involve the epidermis and extend into, but not through, the dermis. Examples are tape burns, sunburns, blisters (unless blood filled, which could indicate deeper tissue damage), some skin tears, and Stage II pressure ulcers (**Figures 2–1** and **2–2**; **Color Plates 1 and 2**).
2. Full-thickness wounds involve a subcutaneous layer or extend into muscle or bone. Examples are deep leg ulcers, deep burns, and Stage III or Stage IV pressure ulcers.

WOUND STAGING

If the wound is a pressure ulcer, you must stage it. It is important to remember that staging is inappropriate until nonviable tissue is removed from the wound bed. Until necrotic tissue is removed and the wound bed is visible, the wound is unstageable (Bergstrom, et al., 1994, p. 18). Once the wound stage is identified,

Figure 2–1 Intact Purple Heel Blister. Suspected deep tissue injury.
Clinical Objectives:
(1) Protect
(2) Relieve pressure
See Color Plate 1.

Figure 2–2 Intact Heel Blister Resolving.
Clinical Objectives:
(1) Protect
(2) Relieve pressure
See Color Plate 2.

the wound should not be backstaged. As a Stage IV pressure ulcer heals, it is a healing Stage IV. Once it is closed, it is a healed Stage IV.

WOUND LOCATION AND DIMENSIONS

The wound location should be precisely identified. Use directional terms like right or left, medial or distal, and the correct anatomical location. A body drawing can be used (**Figure 2–3**).

The dimensions of the wound should be measured and recorded weekly. Measure the length, width, and depth in centimeters. A disposable tape measure can be used.

Measure the length at the longest point on the wound surface, measured head to toe.

Measure the width at the widest point on the wound surface, measured side to side.

To determine a wound's depth, insert a sterile, cotton-tipped applicator into the deepest part of the wound bed, grasp the applicator at skin level, and then measure the applicator from its tip to your fingers.

Figure 2–3 Common Locations for Chronic Wounds.
Source: Courtesy of Knoll Pharmaceuticals, (1999), Mount Olive, NJ.

Wound tunneling (**Color Plate 7**) or undermining (**Color Plate 13**) is measured by inserting a cotton-tipped applicator to measure depth in centimeters. Describe the location using the face of a clock, with 12 o'clock at the patient's head, and 6 o'clock at the patient's feet. Always work in a clockwise direction when documenting the deepest sizes of tunneling or undermining. Example: 2 cm of undermining from 2 o'clock to 6 o'clock.

WOUND BED

Note the status of the wound bed. Document necrotic tissue, fibrin slough, and red granulation tissue. Quantifying the percentage of tissue involved can help paint a picture of the wound bed and facilitate assessment and documentation of changes in the wound bed. Example: The wound bed is 50% black eschar, 25% fibrin slough, and 25% red granulation tissue.

WOUND ODOR

Note the presence or absence of odor. When you detect an odor, note its strength and any identifying characteristics.

WOUND DRAINAGE

Describe any exudate, including the amount, color, and characteristics such as serous, purulent, or viscous. Example: Is the old dressing dry? Is it 25%, 50%, or 100% saturated? How long has it been since the dressing was changed? (See **Table 2–1**.)

TIP Dissolving black eschar/slough is not necessarily infection. Clean the wound then assess for infection.

Table 2–1 Wound Exudate Characteristics

Exudate Type	Color	Consistency	Significance
Sanguineous/bloody	Red	Thin, watery	Indicates new blood vessel growth or disruption of blood vessels
Serosanguineous	Light red to pink	Thin, watery	Normal during inflammatory and proliferative phases of healing
Serous	Clear, light color	Thin, watery	Normal during inflammatory and proliferative phases of healing
Seropurulent	Cloudy, yellow to tan	Thin, watery	May be first signal of impending wound infection
Purulent/pus	Yellow, tan, or green	Thick, opaque	Signals wound infection; may be associated with odor

Source: Reprinted from Bates-Jensen, B. M. (1998). Management of exudate and infection. In C. Sussman & B. M. Bates-Jenkins (Eds.), *Wound care: A collaborative practice manual for physical therapists and nurses* (p. 160). Gaithersburg, MD: Aspen Publishers.

WOUND MARGINS

TIP A plastic sandwich bag can be used for tracing the wound. Place the bag on the wound, and trace the outline of the wound with a permanent, fine-tip marker. Add location markers such as head, feet, and anatomical location. Throw away the side that was touching the wound, and place the clean side with the tracing in the chart.

Assess the extent and depth of undermining and the condition of wound edges. Are the wound edges macerated from too much moisture or rolled under? Are they sharp and distinct or diffuse and irregular? Is epithelial tissue visible around the wound edges? Note the presence or absence of induration.

PERIWOUND SKIN

Assess color, induration, warmth, and edema of the skin around the wound. Redness of the surrounding skin can be indicative of unrelieved pressure. Irritation of the surrounding skin can result from exposure to feces or urine, a reaction to the dressing or tape, or inappropriate removal of dressing or tape. Redness, tenderness, warmth, and swelling are classical clinical signs of infection. (See **Figure 2–4**.)

Figure 2–4 Heel Ulcer with Yellow Slough. Periwound skin macerated due to inappropriate topical treatment.
Clinical Objectives:
(1) Clean
(2) Remove necrotic tissue
(3) Manage exudate
(4) Relieve pressure
See Color Plate 3.

PAIN

Note presence or absence of pain in the wound or periwound area. Use your agency's guidelines for assessing pain.

REFERENCE

Bergstrom, N., et al. (1994). *Treatment of pressure ulcers*. Clinical Practice Guideline No. 15. AHCPR Publication No. 95-0652. Rockville, MD: U.S. Department of Health and Human Services. Public Health Services, Agency for Health Care Policy and Research.

BIBLIOGRAPHY

Buckley, K. M., et al. (2005). The use of digital images in evaluating homecare nurses' knowledge of wound assessment. *Journal of Wound, Ostomy, and Continence Nursing, 32*(5), 307–316.

Cooper, D. (2000). Assessment, measurement, and evaluation: Their pivotal roles in wound healing. In R. Bryant (Ed.), *Acute and chronic wounds: Nursing management* (pp. 51–81). St. Louis, MO: Mosby.

Sussman, C. (1998). Assessment of the skin and wound measurement. In C. Sussman & B. M. Bates-Jensen (Eds.), *Wound care: A collaborative practice manual for physical therapists and nurses* (pp. 49–102). Gaithersburg, MD: Aspen.

Color Plate 1 Intact Purple Heel Blister. Suspected deep tissue injury.

Color Plate 2 Intact Heel Blister Resolving.

Color Plate 3 Heel Ulcer with Yellow Slough. Periwound skin macerated due to inappropriate topical treatment.

Color Plate 4 Eschar on Wound Bed.

Color Plate 5 Autolytic Debridement in Progress: Slough Wound Base.

Color Plate 6 Chest Tube Site with Copious Purulent Drainage on Gauze Packing.

Color Plate 7 Chest Tube Site (Same as Previous Picture) with Large Tunnel.

Color Plate 8 Skin Tear with Hypergranulation Tissue. Note fragile "onion peel" type skin surrounding the wound.

Color Plate 9
Pressure Ulcer on
Sacrum. Unable to
stage due to yellow
necrotic tissue on
the base of the
wound.

Color Plate 10 Stage I Pressure Ulcer.
Nonblanchable erythema.

Color Plate 11 Stage II Pressure Ulcer at Sacral Region. Thin layer-desiccated tissue.

Color Plate 12 Healing Stage III Pressure Ulcer.

Color Plate 13 Stage IV Pressure Ulcer on Sacrum with Necrotic Tissue and Undermining.

Color Plate 14 Arterial Ulcers. Note dry, flaky skin and absence of hair.

Color Plate 15 Ischemic Foot with Gangrene. Do not initiate topical treatment. Notify physician of status and any changes immediately.

healed closed
area

Color Plate 16 Full-Thickness Venous Stasis Ulcer on Dark-Skinned Person. Healed skin will remain light.

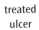

treated
ulcer

ulcer slough
base

Color Plate 17 Venous Stasis Ulcer, Right Medial Ankle. Note edema, gaiter staining, and closed wound on left leg.

Color Plate 18 Venous Stasis Ulcer. Shallow wound bed, irregular shape, wound bed ruddy red with some yellow slough.

Color Plate 19 Ulcer with Mixed Disease. Patient is not a surgical candidate.

Color Plate 20 Neuropathic Ulcer; Charcot Foot.

Color Plate 21 Diabetic Ulcer Needs Saucer-Style Debridement of Callus. Note dry skin at ankle, typical of diabetics.

Color Plate 22 Diabetic Foot Ulcer with Hypergranulation Tissue, Callus Margin.

Color Plate 23 Skin Tear with 75% of Epidermal Flap Missing.

Color Plate 24 Clean, Granular Surgical Wound with Small Amount of Slough in Center. Note colostomy.

Color Plate 25 Open Surgical Incision with Tunneling.

Color Plate 26 Necrotic Tissue (Eschar) at Above-Knee Amputation Site of Stump Incision Line. Note erythema and poorly approximated incision line.

Color Plate 27 Suspected deep tissue injury on a person with dark skin.

PART II

Basics of Wound Management

Normal Healing Process

Pamela Brown

To best understand the normal healing process, the clinician needs to know the structure of the skin (**Figure 3–1**).

STRUCTURES OF THE SKIN

The skin is the largest organ of the body. It consists of two layers: epidermis and dermis.

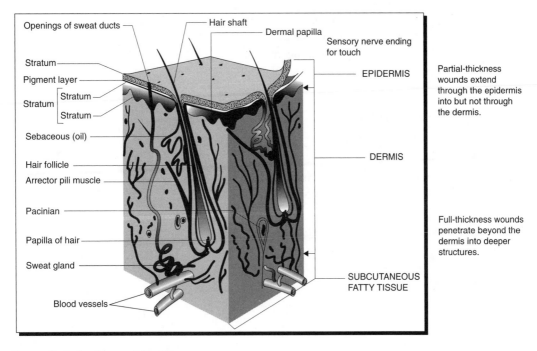

Figure 3–1 Anatomy of the Skin.
Source: Courtesy of Knoll Pharmaceuticals, (1999), Mount Olive, NJ.

Epidermis

The epidermis is the outermost layer of skin. It varies in thickness, but it is usually around 0.1 mm thick with five layers of squamous cells.

Functions

- protection from ultraviolet light and outside contamination
- sensations
- temperature control
- prevention of dehydration
- vitamin D production
- may indicate the emotional state of the patient

Dermis

The dermis is connected to the epidermis by a basement membrane.

Functions

- hair production (hair follicles)
- sensation (nerve endings)
- supplies nourishment (removes waste via capillaries)
- provides elasticity (elastin)
- strength support (collagen)
- sweat production (sweat glands)

Deeper Structures

The subcutaneous tissue is called the hypodermis.

- located below dermis
- provides insulation and protection for organs
- stores energy

Table 3–1 Partial-Thickness and Full-Thickness Skin Loss

Thickness of Skin Loss	Definition	Clinical Examples
Partial-thickness skin loss	Extends through the epidermis, into but not through the dermis	Skin tears, abrasions, tape damage, blisters, perineal dermatitis from incontinence; heals by epidermal resurfacing or epithelialization
Full-thickness skin loss	Extends through the epidermis and the dermis, extending into subcutaneous fat and deeper structures	Donor sites, venous ulcers, arterial/ischemic wounds; surgical wounds; heals by granulation tissue formation and contraction

Source: Sussman, C. (1998). Assessment of the skin and wound. In C. Sussman & B. M. Bates-Jensen (Eds.), *Wound care: A collaborative practice manual for physical therapists and nurses* eds. (p. 54). Gaithersburg, MD: Aspen Publishers.

WOUND HEALING PROCESS

The wound healing process is divided into two categories (see **Table 3–1**).

1. Partial-thickness wounds penetrate the epidermis and may extend into the dermis. They heal by epithelialization; that is, the epithelial cells migrate from the wound edges and any remaining hair follicles to resurface the wound. These wounds are usually moist and painful because of the loss of epidermal covering and exposure of nerve endings.
2. Full-thickness wounds extend beyond the dermis into the subcutaneous tissue. They can also involve muscle, tendon, or bone and heal by filling with granulation tissue, contraction, and epithelialization from the wound edges. The healing process is one of granulation tissue formation and contraction.

Acute wounds progress through a predictable series of events that result in a healed wound. This process can be described as a cascade of events with healing phases that overlap. The final result is a healed wound. In contrast, chronic nonhealing wounds fail to proceed through an orderly and timely healing process.

Table 3–2, gives an overview of the normal healing process for full-thickness wounds.

Table 3–2 Normal Healing Process for Full-Thickness Wounds

	Inflammatory Phase* (1 to 4 days postinjury)	**Proliferation Phase*** (4 to 20 days postinjury)	**Maturation Phase*** (21 days to 2 years postinjury)
Main function	Initial healing cascade; removes debris and prepares for new tissue Pain, redness, swelling, heat	Deposition of connective tissue and collagen cross-linking	Strengthening and reorganizing of collagen fibers
Clinical observations	Serous or serosanguineous drainage	Extracellular matrix, commonly called granulation tissue, fills the wound bed with newly formed collagen and blood vessels. The appearance is beefy red. Epithelial cells migrate across the wound surface from wound margins.	Shrinking, thinning, paling of scar
Physiologic actions	Bacteria are killed. Cellular debris is removed. The wound is prepared for tissue regeneration: • Platelets cause blood clotting. • Vasoconstriction and vasodilation direct blood to where it's needed. • Leukocytes and macrophages engulf and kill bacteria.	Macrophages continue to kill bacteria. Fibroblasts deposit collagen to fill the wound bed. New blood vessels extend into the area (angiogenesis). Myofibroblasts cause the wound to contract.	New tissue continues to grow and develop, and the scar is strengthened. Collagen fibers reorganize and remodel, and wound contraction continues.
Tips	If the patient is immunocompromised, inflammation will be suppressed. Risk of infection will increase, and healing can be delayed. Manage increased moisture that may occur during this phase.	A change from beefy red to dusky pink (with or without an increase in drainage) can be a sign of infection.	Even when the wound is completely healed, only about 80% of tensile strength of normal skin is regained. The patient is at risk for recurrent breakdown.

*These phases overlap and occur as a cascade of healing events. For more detailed information on a cellular level, refer to the bibliography at the end of this chapter.

BIBLIOGRAPHY

Baum, C. L., MD, & Arpey, C. J., MD. (2005). Normal cutaneous wound healing. *Dermatologic Surgery, 31*(6), 674–686.

Cooper, D. (1990). The physiology of wound healing: An overview. In D. Krasner (Ed.), *Chronic wound care: A clinical source book for healthcare professionals* (pp. 1–11). King of Prussia, PA: Health Management Publications.

Doughty, D. B., & Sparks-Defriese, B. (2007). Wound-healing physiology. In R. A. Bryant & D. P. Nix (Eds.), *Acute and chronic wounds, Current management concepts* (3rd ed., pp. 56–81). St. Louis, MO: Mosby Elsevier.

Haimowitz, J., & Margolis, D. (1997). Moist wound healing. In D. Krasner & D. Kane (Eds.), *Chronic wound care: A clinical source book for healthcare professionals* (2nd ed., pp. 49–56). Wayne, PA: Health Management Publications.

Sussman, C. (1998). Wound healing biology and chronic wound healing. In C. Sussman & B. M. Bates-Jensen (Eds.), *Wound care: A collaborative practice manual for physical therapists and nurses* (pp. 31–45). Gaithersburg, MD: Aspen.

Basics of Wound Management

Pamela Brown

Wound healing is a complex process involving many factors. When developing a wound healing treatment plan, the clinician should assess the entire patient. The plan should address causative factors and factors that are known to impede the healing process. Dressings should protect the wound, provide a moist environment, and prevent maceration of wound edges. The goal is to create an environment that promotes wound healing and supports the body in healing itself. It is imperative to reevaluate the healing progress at regular intervals. If a wound shows no healing progress in 2 to 4 weeks, reevaluate the patient and the wound treatment plan. Report your findings to the physician.

CAUSATIVE FACTORS

Reduce or eliminate factors that cause wounds. Failure to reduce or eliminate the cause can result in a nonhealing wound despite appropriate systemic and topical therapy.

Pressure

A pressure ulcer is an area of local tissue trauma usually developing where soft tissue is compressed between a bony prominence and any external surface for prolonged time periods. A pressure ulcer is a sign of local tissue necrosis and death.

Friction

Friction is the resistance generated between two objects as they are moved in opposite directions. Example: Skin can be denuded during repositioning.

Shear

Shear occurs when two surfaces are being moved in opposite directions and they do not slide freely across each other. This causes deformities, kinking, or tearing of vessels in deep tissue. Example: When the head of the bed is up and the patient slides down in bed, the skin and superficial fascia can remain fixed against the bed linen, while the deep fascia and skeleton slide down toward the foot of the bed, causing deep tissue damage.

Circulatory Impairment

Compromised circulation, such as peripheral vascular disease and chronic obstructive pulmonary disease, affect healing at a cellular level. Tissue repair is compromised in the absence of adequate blood supply and/or oxygenation.

Neuropathy

Loss of sensation puts the patient at risk for mechanical, chemical, and thermal trauma. This occurs as a complication of prolonged glucose elevation.

Moisture

Moisture, urine, and feces can cause maceration and overhydration of the epidermis. The skin tissue becomes less tolerant to pressure force.

SYSTEMIC SUPPORT

Provide systemic support for wound healing.

Nutrition and Hydration

Failure to address poor nutritional status will result in a nonhealing wound despite appropriate topical therapy. If a patient is at risk, a registered clinical dietitian should assess the patient as part of a multidisciplinary approach to wound management (**Exhibits 4–1** and **4–2**). Look for:

- patients weighing less than 80% of ideal body weight
- an involuntary weight loss of 10% or greater in 6 months
- serum albumin (a measure of protein available for healing) less than 3.5
- total lymphocyte count less than 1800/mm^3
- prealbumin less than 18

Proper hydration is needed to promote blood flow to affected areas (**Exhibit 4–3**).

Diabetes

Wound healing is impaired in patients with diabetes, and they have an increased incidence of infection. Their plan of care should include strict control of blood glucose levels.

Exhibit 4-1 Skin Integrity and Wound Healing: The Role of Nutrition

It has long been recognized but unappreciated that impaired nutritional status and inadequate dietary intake are risk factors for development of pressure ulcers. A well-balanced diet with adequate carbohydrate, protein, fat, water, vitamins, and minerals is necessary to maintain skin integrity.

Calories, protein, water, vitamin C, and zinc are often emphasized to promote wound healing. However, adequate intake of these nutrients or any nutrient alone does not facilitate healing. Sufficient calories plus all essential nutrients are required.

CALORIES

The body's first priority is adequate energy. When the total amount of calories is too low, protein from both the diet and the patient's muscle stores is used as an energy source, the patient loses weight, and adipose tissue as well as lean body mass are lost.

Every wound patient's calorie needs are different. The caloric goal for patients with wounds is to prevent weight loss from occurring. In underweight patients, a slow steady weight gain will increase the speed of wound healing. The three major nutrients—carbohydrate, protein, and fat—provide calories. Carbohydrates and fats are the preferred energy source for a healing wound.

PROTEIN

Dietary protein is needed for tissue maintenance and repair. Protein depletion impairs wound healing by preventing a desirable wound bed from forming. Repletion of calorie and protein status in undernourished patients is associated with shorter time to heal and improved wound strength. Renal function needs to be evaluated when increasing levels of protein.

WATER

Water is an especially important nutrient for patients with wounds. Dehydration is a risk factor for development of wounds, and the water needs of patients with Stages III and IV pressure ulcers are very high. A good rule of thumb is to be sure that all patients receive a minimum of 1 milliliter (ml) of water for every kilocalorie fed, or about 15 ml of water per pound of body weight per day. Wound patients need at least 2000–2500 ml of water a day (2 quarts or more).

Water and other household beverages are adequate sources of water in most cases and can be given orally or by feeding tube. These fluids, however, are not adequate to replace the fluid and electrolyte losses that accompany vomiting, diarrhea, or other sources of gastrointestinal fluid losses. In these cases, a rehydration solution, such as Equalyte® (Ross Products Division of Abbott Laboratories), which is specifically designed to match and replace these losses, is needed.

VITAMIN C

Because nutritional deficiency has been associated with impaired wound healing, supplemental intake of vitamins and minerals is often thought to be important for wound healing. Although not appropriate for all patients, vitamin and mineral supplements are probably most beneficial for patients with a history of poor intake who are therefore likely to have limited nutrient stores. A general one-a-day type vitamin and mineral supplement equal to 100% of the Reference Daily Intake (RDI) for vitamins and minerals is prudent for patients with wounds.

(continues)

Exhibit 4–1 (*continues*)

Vitamin C is essential in collagen synthesis. Collagen and fibroblasts compose the basis for the structure of a new healing wound bed. A deficiency of vitamin C prolongs healing time, decreases wound strength, and contributes to decreased resistance to infection. There is no evidence, however, that human wound healing is improved by providing doses of vitamin C many times greater than the RDI of from 75 milligrams (mg.) for females to 90 mg. for males per day. It is reasonable to increase vitamin C intake through consumption of fruits, vegetables, and juices for persons with extensive wounds who may rapidly exhaust their body reserves and for those with a history of poor intake.

ZINC

Zinc deficiency can occur through wound drainage or excessive gastrointestinal fluid losses (diarrhea), corticosteroid use, or can be due to long-term low dietary intake. Chronic, severe zinc deficiency results in abnormal function of white blood cells and lymphocytes, increased susceptibility to infection, and delayed wound healing. Large amounts of dietary zinc (above 40mg /d.), however, interfere with copper metabolism and are not advisable. The amount of zinc in a multiple vitamin/mineral supplement is generally adequate. It is much more preferable and safer to provide the RDI for zinc (12–15 mg/day) through a one-a-day type multiple vitamin and mineral supplement than to provide individual zinc supplementation at very high levels (such as zinc sulfate 200–300 mg daily or three times daily).

Source: Courtesy of Ross Products Division of Abbott Laboratories, (2000), Columbus, OH.

Exhibit 4–2 Suggested Diet for Wound Healing

- Calories (energy)—provide enough calories to prevent weight loss, promote wound healing, and prevent infection; 30–35 calories per kilogram (kg) body weight per day.
- Protein—adequate for positive nitrogen balance and to promote new cell development; 1.2–2 g of protein per kg of body weight per day. Optimal protein distribution is to have equal amounts of protein in each meal to maximize protein synthesis.
- Fluid—30 ml per kg body weight per day; adjust per individual need.
- Vitamin/minerals
  - Vitamin C helps make collagen, promotes healing, and helps build resistance to infection.
  - Vitamin A helps make new skin cells.
  - Zinc promotes wound healing and improves immunity.
  - Iron helps carry oxygen to nourish the cells.

Note: Vitamin/mineral supplementation is often recommended if the oral diet is inadequate. If deficiencies are confirmed or suspected, a multivitamin may be used. Due to toxicity and nutrient interactions, multivitamins should not be used in high doses and should only be used if ordered by the physician. See Suggested Nutrient-Rich Foods for Wound Healing in Appendix 4–A and High-Calorie/High-Protein Ideas in Appendix 4–B.

Source: Courtesy of Healthcare Dietary Services, Inc. (1999), Evansville, IN.

Exhibit 4–3 Signs and Symptoms of Dehydration

- If the client/resident is able to drink independently, keep water or other beverages at bedside so that they are easily accessible and in a container that can be handled easily.

- If the client/resident doesn't initiate drinking, offer water each time the client/resident is turned (every 2 hours).

Look for:

- dry skin
- cracked lips
- thirst (may be diminished in the elderly)
- fever
- loss of appetite
- nausea
- dizziness
- increased confusion
- increase in pulse
- constipation (recent diarrhea can explain the dehydrated state, whereas constipation is a common occurrence when dehydration exists)
- concentrated urine

Source: Courtesy of Healthcare Dietary Services, Inc. (1999), Evansville, IN.

Steroid Administration

Steroids are known to inhibit epithelial proliferation and to exert powerful anti-inflammatory effects. Vitamin A can partially counteract the effect of steroids.

Immunosuppression

Any disease process or medication that suppresses the immune system can delay wound healing.

Aging

The aging process produces many changes in the skin that can impede the healing process. It is important to optimize healing and to eliminate any correctable impediments to healing. Optimal systemic and topical support will enhance the healing process.

Obesity and Wound Healing

There are multiple issues to consider for the patient who is morbidly obese. Frequently, these patients have numerous comorbidities complicating their care and their wound care. Some of these comorbidities can include diabetes, cardio-vascular disease, hypertension, and social and psychological stress.

In the home environment, it may be necessary not only to include special equipment, but also to have the environment evaluated to see if the additional equipment can be used safely and effectively. Special consideration must also be given to prevent injury to the caregivers.

In the hospital and nursing home environment, standard equipment weight limits may not provide safety for the patient. Weight limits must be considered for all of the equipment used in the care of the obese patient. Special equipment with weight loads over 500–600 pounds may be required. This can include beds, side rails, lifts, wheelchairs, stretchers, walkers, and toilet facilities.

Issues to consider include:

- nutrition
- mobility
- wound considerations
- pain management

Developing protocols to implement when a morbidly obese patient is admitted to service can provide direction for decision making and care planning. This can be invaluable in preventing complications. For more detailed information, refer to the following resources list and the bibliography at the end of this chapter.

Resources:

- www.hill-rom.com
- www.kcl1.com
- www.sizewiserentals.com

PRINCIPLES OF TOPICAL THERAPY

The goal of topical therapy is to create an environment that supports the healing process.

Remove Necrotic Tissue

Necrotic tissue can be removed in several ways (**Figure 4–1**; **Color Plate 4**). See **Table 4–1**, Debridement Time Frames.

1. Mechanical debridement
   - wet-to-dry gauze moistened with normal saline. This is a nonselective method and may remove healthy tissue as well as necrotic tissue. This

Figure 4–1 Eschar on Wound Bed.

Clinical Objectives:

(1) Remove eschar

(2) Provide moist wound environment

(3) Manage exudate

See Color Plate 4.

method of debridement is used less today than in the past because safer, more effective treatments are available. Another wound care treatment should be used once the wound bed is cleaned of necrotic tissue.

- whirlpool—for removal of thick exudate, slough, or necrotic tissue. It should be discontinued when the wound bed is clear of necrotic tissue.
- wound irrigation. Safe and effective ulcer irrigation pressures range from 4 to 15 psi (pounds per square inch).

2. Enzymatic debridement—ointments used on necrotic tissue to clean the wound bed.

3. Sharp debridement—surgical debridement of necrotic tissue. Use clean, dry dressing for 8 to 24 hours after sharp debridement associated with bleeding. Then resume moist dressings.

4. Autolytic debridement—breakdown of necrotic tissue by the body's wound fluids, which contain natural enzymes. A moisture-retentive dressing can be

Table 4–1 Debridement Time Frames

Necrotic Tissue Type	Debridement Choice	Expected Outcomes	Time Frame Guide	Notes
Eschar	Autolysis	1. Eschar nonadherent to wound edges 2. Necrotic tissue lifting from wound edges 3. Necrotic tissue soft and soggy 4. Color change from black/brown to yellow/tan	14 days	Depending on type of dressing used for autolysis, may proceed at more rapid rate
Eschar	Enzymatic preparations	1. Eschar nonadherent to wound edges 2. Necrotic tissue lifting from wound edges 3. Necrotic tissue soft and soggy 4. Color change from black/brown to yellow/tan 5. Change from eschar to slough	14 days	Requires compliance with dressing changes in order to be effective
Eschar	Sharp	1. Removal/elimination of eschar if done one time or significant change in amount and adherence if sequential	Immediate if one time, 7 days if sequential	If sequential sharp debridement used in conjunction with enzymatic preparation or autolysis, may expect clean wound base in 7 days
Slough or fibrin	Autolysis or enzymatic preparations	1. Necrotic tissue lifting from wound base 2. Necrotic tissue stringy or mucinous 3. Tissue color yellow or white 4. Change in amount of wound covered—gradual decrease to wound predominantly clean	14 days	Will require moderate amount of exudate absorption and protection of surrounding tissues from maceration
Slough or fibrin	Sharp	1. Removal/elimination of necrotic slough if done one time or significant change in amount and adherence if sequential	Immediate if one time, 7 days if sequential	If sequential sharp debridement used in conjunction with enzymatic preparation or autolysis, may expect clean wound base in 7 days
aSASA				

Source: Reprinted from Bates-Jensen, B. M. (1998). Management of necrotic tissue. In C. Sussman & B. M. Bates-Jensen (Eds.) *Wound care: A collaborative practice manual for physical therapists and nurses* (p. 149). Gaithersburg, MD: Aspen Publishers.

used for autolytic debridement. Use with caution and do not use on infected wounds (**Figure 4–2; Color Plate 5).**

- transparent film dressings
- hydrogel dressings
- hydrocolloid dressings

See Debridement Choices for Chronic Wounds at the end of this chapter.

Identify and Eliminate Infection

All wounds are colonized with bacteria. Healing may be impaired if bacterial levels exceed 100,000 per gram of tissue or if the patient has osteomyelitis. Colonization may be minimized through effective wound cleansing and debridement. Proper cleansing of the wound is one of the most effective and most often

Figure 4–2 Autolytic Debridement in Progress: Slough Wound Base.

Clinical Objectives:

(1) Clean

(2) Remove slough

(3) Keep moist

(4) Relieve pressure

See Color Plate 5.

overlooked ways to keep the bacterial level down in a wound. Use minimal mechanical force when cleaning a wound with gauze, cloth, or sponges. Traumatized wounds are more susceptible to infection and are slower to heal. Healthy tissue can be damaged. Normal saline is the preferred cleansing agent because it will not harm healing tissue, and it adequately cleans most wounds. If the pressure is too high, it can damage healing tissue. If irrigation pressures are too low, they will not cleanse the wound properly. Safe and effective irrigation pressures of 4 to 15 psi can be obtained using a 19-gauge needle or angiocath with a 35-ml syringe. Pressurized saline designed for wound cleansing is also available (See **Table 4–2** and **Exhibit 4–4**). Signs and symptoms of infection include:

> **TIP** **TIP FOR EFFECTIVE IRRIGATION**
> Pressurized saline designed for wound cleansing and irrigation is available without a prescription at drug stores. A can will provide sterile saline for multiple wound cleansings.

- a wound that does not progress toward healing despite optimal care for 2 to 4 weeks
- increased drainage with or without foul odor
- purulent drainage (thick green or yellow)
- redness or warmth around wound
- cellulitis of surrounding tissue
- pain

Treat Localized Infection

For localized signs of infection, or wounds that do not show progress toward healing after 2 to 4 weeks of optimum care, a 2-week trial of silver composite or topical antibiotic should be considered. Do not use topical antiseptics such as povidone iodine, hydrogen peroxide, or alcohol to decrease bacteria in wound tissue. Numerous studies have shown these antiseptics to be toxic to healing tissue. If no improvement is seen, quantitative bacterial cultures may be ordered. Swab cultures are of questionable value because they detect only the surface contaminants and may not truly reflect the organism(s) causing the infection. However, they may be ordered by the physician if clinical signs of infection are present.

> **TIP** **TIP FOR SWAB CULTURE**
> First, cleanse the wound with normal saline. Swab the wound bed using a Z technique. Pressure is applied to the swab to cause tissue/fluid to be absorbed in the swab. Place the swab in the appropriate container immediately and transport it to the lab.

Treat Systemic Infection

For systemic signs of infection, such as fever, chills, weakness, or increased heart rate, the patient should be evaluated immediately for bacteremia, sepsis, advancing cellulitis, or osteomyelitis and treated with the appropriate antibiotic.

Table 4–2 Comparison of Wound Characteristics in Inflamed and Infected Wounds

Wound Characteristic	Inflamed Wounds	Infected Wounds
Erythema (redness or purple-gray color)	Usually presents with well-defined borders. Not as intense in color. May be seen as skin discoloration in dark-skinned persons, such as a purple or gray hue to the skin or a deepening of normal ethnic color.	Edges of erythema or skin discoloration may be diffuse and indistinct. May present as very intense erythema or discoloration with well-demarcated and distinct borders. Red stripes streaking up or down from the area indicate infection.
Elevated temperature	Usually noted as increase in temperature at wound site and surrounding tissues.	Systemic fever (may not be present in older adult populations).
Exudate: odor	Any odor present may be due to necrotic tissue in the wound, solubilization of necrotic tissue, or the type of wound therapy in use, not necessarily infection.	Specific odors are related to some bacterial organisms, such as the sweet smell of Pseudomonas or the ammonia odor associated with Proteus.
Exudate: amount	Usually minimal; if injury is recent, you should see a gradual decrease in exudate amount over 3–5 days.	Usually moderate to large amounts; if injury is recent, you will not see a decrease in exudate amount—the amount remains high or increases.
Exudate: character	Bleeding and serosanguineous to serous.	Serous and seropurulent to purulent.
Pain	Variable.	Pain is persistent and continues for an unusual amount of time. Take wound etiology and subjective nature of pain into account when assessment is performed.
Edema and induration	May be slight swelling or firmness at wound edge.	May indicate infection if edema and indurations are localized and accompanied by warmth.

Source: Reprinted from Bates-Jensen, B. M. (1998). Management of necrotic tissue. In C. Sussman & B. M. Bates-Jensen (Eds.), *Wound care: A collaborative practice manual for physical therapists and nurses* (pp. 151–156, Appendix 7-A). Gaithersburg, MD: Aspen Publishers.

Exhibit 4–4 Proper Procedures for Cleaning Wounds

SHALLOW WOUND CLEANSING PROCEDURE

Supplies

- clean, shallow container
- saltwater solution or wound cleanser solution
- gauze
- catch basin
- wound dressing

Procedure

1. Follow universal precautions regarding handwashing, gloving, and protection from splashing.

2. Warm the saltwater solution or wound cleanser solution to lukewarm. Test the temperature with your elbow.

3. Pour the amount of solution you expect to use into a clean, shallow container. Then the balance of the solution will remain clean.

4. Moisten a pad of clean gauze dressing (bandage) with the solution in the clean, shallow container.

5. Place the catch basin under the wound edge to collect the fluid.

6. Work in a circular pattern, starting at the center of the wound, to gently cleanse the wound with the moistened gauze. Work outward toward the edge of the wound and surrounding skin. Remove any pus or loose tissue with the gauze pad. Do not press hard or scrub because this will damage the tissue and slow healing. Do not return to the wound center after cleansing. This will recontaminate the wound.

7. Discard the moist gauze and any unused solution in the container.

8. Apply the prescribed dressing (bandage) as directed.

Helpful hint: Keep the patient and the room warm while cleansing the wound. The patient will be more comfortable. Cooling will slow the healing of the wound.

DEEP WOUND CLEANSING PROCEDURE

Deep wounds often have tunnels that run under the skin. Pus and dead tissue trapped in these tunnels are sources for infection. These tunnels can be cleansed by using a syringe filled with saltwater solution to flush them.

SUPPLIES

- 35-ml size syringe
- saltwater solution
- gauze
- catch basin
- towels
- wound dressing

PROCEDURE

1. Follow universal precautions regarding handwashing, gloving, and protection from splashing.

2. Warm the saltwater solution to lukewarm. Test the temperature with your elbow.

3. Fill a 35-ml syringe with warm saltwater solution.

4. Place a catch basin and clean towels under the wound edge to collect the fluid.

5. Insert the tip end of the syringe into the tunnel and squirt fluid into the tunnel. Put in the entire amount of the solution that is in the syringe. Repeat three times or until the fluid that comes out is clear, whichever occurs last.

6. Following the running out of the solution, gently massage the tissues with your fingers to express extra fluid.

7. After the wound is cleansed, loosely pack it with dressing materials as prescribed. This will help to prevent infection from traveling up the tunnel.

8. The dirty fluid collected in the basin should be flushed down the toilet.

Helpful hint: Keep the patient and the room warm while cleansing the wound. This will make the patient more comfortable. Cooling will slow the healing of the sore.

Source: Courtesy of Kaiser Permanente, Southern California Regional Health Education, (1999), Los Robles, CA.

Pack Dead Space

Open cavities provide a collection space for wound exudate, which can be a medium for bacterial growth and abscess formation. Open cavities, including sinus tracts, should be loosely packed to absorb drainage and prevent superficial wound closure over a fluid-filled defect (**Figures 4–3** and **4–4; Color Plates 6** and **7**).

Control Odor

Odor can be caused by bacteria in the necrotic wound tissue and by an accumulation of drainage. Management of odor can be achieved through adjusting the frequency of dressing changes and appropriate cleansing with each dressing change. Debridement of necrotic tissue and use of antimicrobials may help. In some instances charcoal dressings also can be used to manage wound odor.

Absorb Excess Exudate

Large amounts of exudate can macerate periwound skin.

Figure 4–3 Chest Tube Site with Copious Purulent Drainage on Gauze Packing.
Clinical Objectives:
(1) Clean
(2) Manage exudate
(3) Loosely pack dead space
(4) Culture if appropriate
See Color Plate 6.

Maintain Moist Wound Surface

A moist wound surface facilitates wound healing. Choose a dressing that keeps the surrounding intact skin dry while keeping the wound bed moist.

Protect Against Heat and Cold

Epidermal migration is enhanced when normal body temperature is maintained.

Protect the Healing Wound

Healing tissue is very fragile, and a dressing should protect it from trauma and invasion.

Figure 4–4 Chest Tube Site (Same as Previous Figure) with Large Tunnel.
Clinical Objectives:
(1) Clean
(2) Pack wound loosely
(3) Manage exudate
See Color Plate 7.

Pain

All patients should be assessed for pain. If they are experiencing pain, the etiology must be determined. Is the pain related to the disease process or the treatment? Once the etiology is determined, interventions can be planned, such as covering the wound, adjusting support services, and repositioning. Analgesics should be provided as needed.

CLEAN, NO-TOUCH WOUND CARE IN THE HOME

Handwashing is the single most important means of preventing the spread of infection.

For the treatment of pressure ulcers, the Agency for Healthcare Research and Quality states: "Clean dressings, as opposed to sterile ones, are recommended for home use until research demonstrates otherwise. This recommendation is in keeping with principles regarding nosocomial infections, and with past success of clean urinary catheterization in the home setting, and takes into account the expense of sterile dressings and the dexterity required to apply them" (Bergstrom, et al., 1994, p. 65). The no-touch technique can be used for dressing changes. This technique is a method of changing surface dressings without touching the wound or the surface of any dressing that might be in contact with the wound. In conjunction with this technique, a clean field is prepared, clean gloves are worn to remove the dressing, and a new pair of gloves is donned to apply the new dressing. Steps are included to prevent direct contamination of material and supplies. Many agencies use a no-touch technique. Follow your agency's policy.

WOUND CARE SOLUTIONS YOU CAN MIX AT HOME

Normal saline is a safe, effective, noncytotoxic solution that is used for wound cleansing.

Dakin's solution and acetic acid should not be routinely used in wound care. Studies have shown that they are cytotoxic to wounds. However, there may be circumstances when they can be used for a short period of time, and a physician orders them. These solutions can be prepared in the home. Use your agency's policy for clean versus sterile preparation. The following chart describes how to make these solutions in the home. Label all containers. The solution is stable for 24 hours from date of preparation.

Solution	Ingredients
0.9% normal saline	4 cups sterile water,* 2 tsp salt (iodized or noniodized table salt)
.025% acetic acid	5 cups sterile water, 4 tbsp white distilled vinegar
Dakin's solution	
Full strength (0.50)	1 pint sterile water, 50 ml bleach
Half strength (0.25)	1 pint sterile water, 25 ml bleach
Quarter strength (0.125)	1 pint sterile water, 12.5 ml bleach

*To prepare sterile water, boil water for 20 minutes.

CASE STUDY

Mrs. Jones is an 84-year-old woman who lives with her husband in a single-family home. She has a diagnosis of dementia. Her husband is the primary caregiver and is 86 years old. Four months ago her condition deteriorated, and her husband was no longer able to get her out of bed. He began using diapers to manage incontinence and fed her small meals five or six times a day. He hired a caregiver who came for 4 hours 2 mornings a week.

After 3 months in bed, Mrs. Jones developed a pressure ulcer on her sacrum. For 1 month, Mr. Jones provided wound care using home remedies. To his untrained eye, the wound was not getting better. He notified the physician, and arrangements were made for a home visit by the

CASE STUDY

doctor. After the visit, the doctor ordered wound care of gauze moistened with normal saline twice a day and a home health evaluation.

The RN case manager assessed the wound as a Stage III pressure sore with enough depth to need packing. The wound measured 3 centimeters (cm) long, 2 cm wide, and 1.5 cm deep. The wound bed was 100% red granulation tissue. There was a moderate amount of serous drainage. The wound edges were intact. There were no signs or symptoms of infection. The RN recommended the following plan:

1. lab work to assess Mrs. Jones's nutritional status (Her serum albumin was 3.5.)
2. a Foley catheter to manage urinary incontinence
3. bed pads instead of diapers
4. a hospital bed with a standard mattress and an overlay for pressure redistribution (After 1 month, if no improvement is seen, the support service can be upgraded to a Group 2 replacement mattress.)
5. skilled nurses three times a week to teach the caregiver how to care for a bedbound, total care patient

TIP With limited nursing visits available, it is imperative to have a plan of care in place as soon as possible. Caregivers must be included in the plan so that they will be able to provide the care when nursing is not available.

After 1 month, the wound was improving, and Mr. Jones had been instructed in his wife's care. Skilled nurses were then reduced to once a week to assess wound healing progress and to change the Foley catheter monthly. The Foley will be discontinued when the wound is healed.

REFERENCE

Bergstrom, N., et al. (1994). *Treatment of pressure ulcers*. Clinical Practice Guideline No. 15. AHCPR Publication No. 95-0652. Rockville, MD: U.S. Department of Health and Human Services. Public Health Services, Agency for Health Care Policy and Research.

BIBLIOGRAPHY

Alvarez, O., et al. (1990). Principles of moist wound healing: Indications for chronic wounds. In D. Krasner (Ed.), *Chronic wound care: A clinical source book for health care professionals* (pp. 266–281). King of Prussia, PA: Health Management Publications.

Cornwell, P., et al. (2010). The use of Dakin's solution in chronic wounds. *Journal of Wound, Ostomy, and Continence Nursing, 37*(1), 94–103.

Doughty, D. B. (1992). Principles of wound healing and wound management. In R. Bryant (Ed.), *Acute and chronic wounds: Nursing management* (pp. 1–25). St. Louis, MO: Mosby-Year Book.

Evans, E. (2005). Nutritional assessment in chronic wound care. *Journal of Wound, Ostomy, and Continence Nursing, 32*(5), 317–320.

Murphy, K., & Gallagher, S. (2001). Options in practice: Care of an obese patient with an ulcer. *Journal of Wound, Ostomy, and Continence Nursing, 28*(3), 171–176.

Rolstad, B. S., & Ovington, L. G. (2007). Principles of wound management. In R. Bryant & D. Nix (Eds.), *Acute and chronic wounds: Current management concepts* (3rd ed., pp. 391–426). St. Louis, MO: Mosby.

Sussman, C., & Bates-Jensen, B. (Eds.). (1998). *Wound care: A collaborative practice manual for physical therapists and nurses.* Gaithersburg, MD: Aspen.

Suggested Nutrient-Rich Foods for Wound Healing

FOODS RICH IN PROTEIN

- beef
- chicken
- pork
- turkey
- fish
- beans
- milk
- cheese
- ice cream
- peanut butter
- eggs
- nuts
- cottage cheese
- yogurt

FOODS RICH IN VITAMIN C

- oranges
- orange juice
- grapefruit
- broccoli
- lemons
- cantaloupe
- green pepper
- strawberries
- kale
- cabbage
- tomatoes
- turnip greens
- juices with vitamin C added

FOODS RICH IN VITAMIN A

- liver
- egg yolks
- broccoli
- kale
- greens
- apricots
- cantaloupe
- sweet potatoes
- whole milk
- fortified skim or low-fat milk
- carrots
- spinach

FOODS RICH IN ZINC

- shellfish
- oatmeal
- rice
- eggs
- nuts
- organ meats (liver, heart, gizzard)
- dried beans and peas
- yogurt

FOODS RICH IN IRON

- liver
- beef
- pork
- beans

- spinach
- peanuts
- sardines
- tuna
- dried fruit

- egg yolks
- oysters
- enriched bread/cereals with iron
- raisins

Combine iron-rich foods or supplement with vitamin C–rich foods for best absorption.

High-Calorie/High-Protein Ideas

GOALS

- to eat enough calories to prevent protein from being used as energy instead of for tissue building
- to provide enough calories and protein to reach and maintain goal weight

SUGGESTIONS

Cheese

Melt on sandwiches, meats, fish, vegetables, and eggs. Grate in sauces, casseroles, mashed potatoes, rice, pastas, and breads. Stuff into vegetables and meatloaf. Spread cream cheese on sandwiches, sliced fruit, and crackers. Mix cottage cheese in pastas, gelatins, pancake batter, and egg dishes.

Whole Milk/Cream

Add or substitute for water in food preparation. Serve cream sauces on vegetables, eggs, pastas, or rice. Pour cream on cereals, fruits, desserts. Top desserts, fruits, molded salads, and hot beverages with whipped cream.

Powdered Milk

Blend 1 cup powdered milk into 1 quart whole milk to make it higher in protein and calories. Add powder to meatloaf, casseroles, sauces, cream soups, and shakes.

Ice Cream/Yogurt

Spread between cookies, cake slices, or graham crackers. Blend into shakes, sodas. Add to cereals, fruits, gelatins, desserts, and pies. Top with fruit, nuts, syrups, sauces, whipped cream, and nut butters.

Eggs

Top salads, vegetables, casseroles, soups, stews, pastas, and potatoes with chopped, hard-cooked eggs. Add pasteurized egg substitute into mashed potatoes, vegetable purées, shakes, and malts. Do not consume raw eggs.

Nuts/Nut Butter

Spread nut butters on sandwiches, toast, muffins, crackers, fruit slices, pancakes, and waffles. Use as a dip for raw vegetables and fruit. Add to meatloaf, cookies, bread, muffins, vegetables, and salads. Blend nut butters with milk drinks or swirl through ice cream and yogurt. Top cookies or cakes with nut butters. Serve nuts as snacks. Roll bananas in chopped nuts.

Meat/Fish

Use in omelets, soufflés, quiches, sandwich fillings, and poultry stuffing. Add small pieces to vegetable salads, casseroles, soups, stuffed baked potatoes, and biscuit ingredients. Wrap in pie crust or biscuit dough as turnovers.

Peas/Beans

Add cooked dry peas and beans or tofu to soups, pastas, casseroles, and meat or milk-based dishes. Mash with cheese and milk. Add textured vegetable protein to burgers, meatloaf, spaghetti sauce, casseroles, and sandwich filling.

ADDITIONAL TIPS

You don't always have to eat a lot, but try to eat often. Try using liquid nutritional supplements between meals to help increase your nutritional intake. (They are available in grocery stores and drug stores.)

To increase calories, drink fruit juice instead of water. Double or triple the portion sizes of added fats and oils (butter, margarine, cream cheese, sour cream, avocado). If not enough protein can be taken in foods, consider granular protein supplements. These can be added to food, given between meals or with medications.

SNACKS

Try to eat six times a day, or every 2 to 3 hours. Watch the clock! Eat, even if you are not hungry.

250-CALORIE SNACKS

- 8 buttery style crackers, 1 oz cheddar cheese, or 1 tbs peanut butter
- ½ sandwich: 1 slice bread, 2 oz cheese or meat, 1 tsp mayonnaise
- quesadilla: 1 tortilla, 2 oz cheese, salsa
- whole apple (sliced) with 2 tbs peanut butter
- 1 cup pudding or fruit yogurt
- 1 slice pizza with extra cheese
- 1 cup whole milk mixed with 1/3 cup dry skim milk powder
- 8-oz can liquid nutritional supplement providing 1 calorie per ml (250 calories/8-oz serving)

350-CALORIE SNACKS

- 10 buttery style crackers, 2 oz cheddar cheese, or 2 tbs peanut butter
- ½ sandwich: 1 slice bread, 2 oz meat or cheese, 2 tsp mayonnaise, 1 slice avocado
- 1 tortilla, 2 oz cheese, salsa, with 1 cup orange juice
- whole banana with 2 tbs peanut butter
- 1 envelope instant breakfast made with whole milk
- shake made with 1 cup whole milk and 1/2 cup ice cream
- 1 carton regular yogurt (not low fat), with 1/3 cup granola or trail mix
- 8-oz can liquid nutritional supplement providing 1.5 calories per ml (350 calories/8-oz serving)

Debridement Choices for Chronic Wounds

Wound Type	Tissue Type	Consistency	Adherence	Amount of Debris	Debridement Choices	Rationale and Notes
Pressure sores	Black/brown eschar	Hard	Firmly adherent, attached to all edges and base of wound	75%–100% of wound covered	1. *Autolytic*—best choice is transparent film dressing. May use hydrocolloid or hydrogel; score eschar with scalpel for more rapid results. 2. *Enzymatic ointment with secondary dressing*—must score eschar with scalpel.	1. Transparent film dressings trap fluid at the wound surface with no absorptive capabilities, providing for more rapid hydration of the eschar and facilitating autolysis. Hydrocolloid/hydrogel dressings have an absorptive capacity and may require more time for autolysis. 2. Enzymatic ointments effective against collagen and protein may be most effective.
	Black/brown eschar or Yellow/tan slough	Soft, stringy Soft, soggy	Adherent, attached to wound base; may or may not be attached to wound edges	50%–100% of wound covered	1. *Autolytic*—best choices are hydrocolloids and hydrogels; composite dressings may also be beneficial. 2. *Enzymatic ointment with secondary dressing.*	1. Hydrocolloids and hydrogels provide for absorption of mild to moderate amounts of exudate while maintaining a wound environment to facilitate autolysis.

Wound Type	Tissue Type	Consistency	Adherence	Amount of Debris	Debridement Choices	Rationale and Notes
Pressure sores (continued)					3. *Sharp, sequential, or one time* —may be used alone or in conjunction with any of the above methods.	2. Enzymatic ointments effective against collagen and protein may be most effective. May need to protect intact skin from enzyme and excess exudate.
	Yellow/tan slough	Soft, stringy	Adherent, attached to wound base, may or may not be attached to wound edges or loosely adherent to wound base	Less than 50% of wound covered	1. *Autolytic*—best choices are hydrocolloids and hydrogels. 2. *Enzymatic ointment with secondary dressing.* 3. *Sharp, sequential, or one time* —may be used alone or in conjunction with any of the above methods.	1. Hydrocolloids and hydrogels provide for absorption of mild to moderate amounts of exudate while maintaining a moist wound environment to facilitate autolysis. 2. Enzymatic ointments effective against collagen and protein may be most effective. May need to protect intact skin from enzyme and excess exudate.

(continues)

Wound Type	Tissue Type	Consistency	Adherence	Amount of Debris	Debridement Choices	Rationale and Notes
Pressure sores (continued)	Yellow slough	Mucinous	Loosely adherent to wound base, clumps scattered throughout wound	50%–100% of wound covered	1. *Autolytic*—best choices are hydrocolloids and hydrogels. 2. *Enzymatic ointment with secondary dressing.*	1. Hydrocolloids and hydrogels provide for absorption of mild to moderate amounts of exudate while maintaining a moist wound environment to facilitate autolysis. 2. Enzymatic ointments effective against collagen and protein may be most effective. May need to protect intact skin from enzyme and excess exudate. Should be discontinued when wound is predominantly clean.
Venous disease ulcers	Black/brown eschar	Hard	Firmly adherent, attached to all edges and base of wound	50%–100% of wound covered	1. *Autolytic*—best choices are hydrocolloids and hydrogels. 2. *Enzymatic ointment with secondary dressing.*	1. Hydrocolloids and hydrogel dressings have absorptive capacity, which helps prevent maceration of surrounding tissues and promotes autolysis. 2. Enzymatic ointments effective against fibrin may be most effective.

Wound Type	Tissue Type	Consistency	Adherence	Amount of Debris	Debridement Choices	Rationale and Notes
Venous disease ulcers (continued)	Yellow slough	Soft, soggy, or fibrinous	Firmly adherent, attached to all edges and base of wound	50%–100% of wound covered	1. *Autolytic*—best choice are hydrocolloids and hydrogels. 2. *Enzymatic ointment with secondary dressing.* 3. *Sharp, sequential, or one time*—may be used alone or in conjunction with any of the above methods.	1. Hydrocolloids and hydrogel dressings have absorptive capacity, which helps prevent maceration of surrounding tissues and promotes autolysis. 2. Enzymatic ointments effective against fibrin may be most effective. May need to protect intact skin from enzyme and excess exudate. Should be discontinued when wound is predominantly clean.

(continues)

Wound Type	Tissue Type	Consistency	Adherence	Amount of Debris	Debridement Choices	Rationale and Notes
Venous disease ulcers (continued)	Yellow slough	Fibrinous or mucinous	Loosely adherent Clumps scattered throughout wound	Any amount of wound covered	1. *Autolytic*—best choices are hydrocolloids and hydrogels. 2. *Enzymatic ointment with secondary dressing.*	1. Hydrocolloids and hydrogel dressings have absorptive capacity, which helps prevent maceration of surrounding tissues and promotes autolysis. 2. Enzymatic ointments effective against fibrin may be most effective. May need to protect intact skin from enzyme and excess exudate. Should be discontinued when wound is predominantly clean.
Neurotrophic/ diabetic ulcers	White/gray	Hard	Hyperkeratosis, callus formation at wound edges	Involves all/partial wound edges	1. *Sharp, sequential, or one time*—saucerization or callus removal. 2. *Autolytic*—best choices are hydrocolloids and hydrogels.	1. Saucerization may be required at each dressing change. 2. Hydrocolloids and hydrogels soften the callus formation, and this may facilitate dressing removal.

Extreme caution should be taken when caring for patients with ischemic ulcers on lower extremities. See Chapter 7.

Wound Treatments

Donna Oddo

There is no "magic" dressing. Wound dressings are but one component of the formula necessary to heal a patient's wound. It is always necessary to assess the whole patient, treat the underlying cause of the wound, and support wound healing with careful attention to all factors that can delay healing.

Selection of an appropriate wound dressing can be challenging. Health care and wound care are undergoing constant change, and nurses must educate themselves on the principles of wound healing as well as new products. The most common topical treatments are presented in this chapter. The examples provided are not inclusive of all available products, and no endorsement is intended or implied.

To determine the appropriate topical treatment, the clinician must assess the wound bed, wound drainage, depth of tissue damage, presence of infection, and the type and location of the wound. These characteristics will help determine the overall goal of treatment. (**Table 5–1** and **Figure 5–1** will help the clinician choose the appropriate wound care. **Exhibit 5–1** gives guidelines for teaching wound care to patients and caregivers.)

TIP In the home setting, all topical treatments require a physician's order. (See Exhibit 5–3 for "Nuggets from Experience." See Appendix 5–A for information on contacting manufacturers about products.)

TRADITIONAL GAUZE DRESSINGS

Gauze dressings may be nonadherent, woven, or nonwoven. They are moderately absorptive, inexpensive, and easily available. They can be combined with topical agents or other types of dressings. They can cover or fill a wound. They can be loosely packed into tunneling wounds and fluffed for maximum absorption capacity. When applied as a wet-to-dry dressing, they can facilitate debridement. When applied as a wet-to-moist or damp dressing, they act as moisture-retentive dressings. Gauze is available (sterile, nonsterile, in bulk, and with or without an adhesive border).

Table 5–1 Topical Treatment Options

Wound Type (Color/Exudate)	Goal	Wound Depth	
		Superficial	Cavity
Black/low exudate	Rehydrate and loosen eschar. Enhance autolytic debridement.	Hydrogels Hydrocolloids Transparent films Enzymatic debriders	
Yellow/high exudate	Remove slough and absorb exudate.	Hydrocolloids Alginates Enzymes Hydrofiber Foam	Hydrogels Moist packing gauze Enzymes Alginates Hydrofiber Collagen
Yellow/low exudate	Remove slough, absorb exudate, and maintain a moist environment.	Hydrogels Sheet hydrogels Hydrocolloids Transparent film	Hydrogels Impregnated gauze Moist packing gauze Alginates Enzymes
Red/high exudate	Maintain moist environment, absorb exudate, and promote granulation and epithelialization.	Foam Alginates Hydrofibers	Alginates Hydrofiber Moist packing gauze
Red/low exudate	Maintain moist environment and promote granulation and epithelialization.	Hydrocolloids Foam Sheet hydrogels Transparent films	Hydrogels Moist packing gauze
Pink/low exudate	Maintain moist environment and protect and insulate.	Foams Transparent films Hydrocolloids (thin) Nonadherent dressing	
Red, unbroken skin	Prevent skin breakdown.	Hydrocolloids Transparent films	

Source: Adapted from Sussman, C., & Bates-Jensen, B. M. (1998). *Wound care: A collaborative practice manual for physical therapists and nurses.* Gaithersburg, MD: Aspen Publishers.

Purpose

1. cleansing
2. packing
3. covering
4. debriding

Absorbency

Depending upon the design of the dressing, light to moderate.

Figure 5–1 Skin Tear with Hypergranulation Tissue. Note fragile "onion peel" type skin surrounding the wound.

Clinical Objectives:
(1) Clean wound and surrounding skin
(2) Protect wound and surrounding skin
(3) Manage exudate
(4) Manage hypergranulation tissue
See Color Plate 8.

Uses

1. Stage II–IV pressure ulcers
2. lower extremity ulcers
3. surgical wounds
4. infected wounds

Cautions

1. Do not use on skin tears.
2. Avoid using on most graft sites.

Examples

- Curity Cover Sponges (Kendall)
- Curity Gauze Sponges (Kendall)

Exhibit 5–1 Teaching Guide for Topical Treatments*

	Instructions Given (Date/Initials)	Demonstration or Review of Materials (Date/Initials)	Return Demonstration or States Understanding (Date/Initials)
1. Type of Wound			
2. Types of Wound Dressings			
a. Alginate			
b. Films			
c. Foams			
d. Gauze			
e. Hydrogel			
f. Hydrocolloid			
3. Reason for Dressing			
a. Maintain dryness			
b. Add moisture			
c. Retain moisture			
d. Absorb moisture			
4. Wound Care			
a. Demonstrates ability to cleanse a wound			
b. Demonstrates ability to apply a wound dressing and topical agents			
c. Demonstrates ability to protect surrounding skin from maceration			
d. Demonstrates ability to make and record simple wound measurements			
5. Infection Prevention			
a. Demonstrates proper handwashing before and after handling soiled dressings			
b. Understands universal precautions			
c. Knows how to dispose of infectious waste			
d. Recognizes/describes warning signs of local infection: pain, swelling, pus, and warmth			
e. Recognizes signs of systemic infection: lethargy, confusion, elevated temperature			
f. Understands when to call the health care professional if infection is suspected			

	Instructions Given (Date/Initials)	Demonstration or Review of Materials (Date/Initials)	Return Demonstration or States Understanding (Date/Initials)

6. Wound Drainage and Tissue Types
  a. Recognizes and reports accurately the amount of wound drainage
  b. Recognizes tissue types and goals:
    black (dry) = dead → soften, clean
    yellow/tan (soft) = dead → clean
    red/pink (moist) = healthy → protect			

7. Universal Precautions
  a. Handwashing
  b. Use of gloves and protective equipment during care procedures
  c. Disposal of contaminated materials			

8. Wound Cleansing
  a. Shallow wound: cleanse gently from center to edge with saline
  b. Deep wound: uses syringe to flush and then gently massages out extra fluids			

9. When to Notify the Health Care Provider
  a. Signs and symptoms of infection
  b. Failure to improve
  c. Presence of odor
  d. Pus (drainage)
  e. Large amount of pus (drainage)
  f. Elevated temperature or signs of confusion in the older adult			

10. Will Make Appointment to Return for Follow-up Care			

*Must be individualized for each patient and caregiver.

Source: Reprinted from Bates-Jensen, B. M. 1998. Management of exudate and infection. In C. Sussman & B. M. Bates-Jensen (Eds.), *Wound care: A collaborative practice manual for physical therapists and nurses* (pp. 175–176). Gaithersburg, MD: Aspen Publishers.

- Carrington Bordered Gauze (Carrington Laboratories, Inc.)
- Kerlex (Kendall)
- Medline Gauze Sponges (Medline Industries, Inc.)

TIPS
- Use high-quality 100% cotton, tightly woven, 12-ply gauze.
- To pack wounds, gauze should be opened, fluffed, and loosely packed, obliterating dead space but allowing room for absorption and expansion. For deep wounds, only one long dressing piece should be used. If several small dressing pieces are used, one may be left behind when dressing changes are made, which can lead to infection in the wound.
- A wet-to-dry dressing is one in which the gauze is moistened, placed into tunnels or undermined areas or applied to the wound, and allowed to dry. The dressing is then removed dry, without moistening the dressing on removal (in wet, out dry) to debride necrotic tissue.

IMPREGNATED GAUZES

Purpose

Gauzes can be impregnated with a variety of substances including petroleum, sodium chloride, and antiseptics to achieve a variety of healing goals. Most impregnated gauzes are designed to promote a moist healing environment and to facilitate ease in dressing removal without disruption of healing tissue. (See Appendix 5–A.) They are nonadherent and require a secondary dressing.

Absorbency

1. moderate (most)
2. high (crystalline sodium chloride)

Uses

Refer to Table 5–1 to match kinds of impregnated gauzes to wound types. Impregnated gauzes can be used on the following kinds of wounds:

1. Stage II–IV pressure ulcers
2. lower extremity ulcers
3. surgical wounds
4. skin tears (moist products only)
5. grafts
6. infected wounds (particularly crystalline sodium chloride)

Caution

Crystalline sodium chloride is inappropriate for dry wounds.

Examples

- Absorb-A-Salt™ (Dumex Medical)
- ADAPTIC™ (Johnson & Johnson Medical)
- Xeroform Petrolatum Gauze (Kendall)
- Mesalt® (Mölnlycke)
- Vaseline Gauze Dressing (Kendall)
- Dermagran Hydraphillic Wound Dressing (Derma Sciences)
- AMD gauze™ (Kendall)

TIPS
- Always follow manufacturer's recommendations for use and frequency of change.
- Nonadherent impregnated gauze may be refrigerated and may help to decrease pain at the wound site.

ALGINATES

Alginates are composed of natural polysaccharide fibers or are derived from seaweed. They are composed of soft, nonwoven fibers shaped as rope or pads. Alginates are highly absorbent and conform to the shape of the wound. When placed into a wound, an alginate generally interacts with wound exudate to form a gel that maintains a moist healing environment. There must be enough exudate in the wound to convert the dry alginate fibers into a gel. They can require a secondary dressing.

Purpose

1. packing (fills dead space)
2. absorption (absorbs up to 20 times its weight)
3. maintaining moist environment (forms a gel within the wound and facilitates autolytic debridement)

Absorbency

Alginates have moderate to high absorbency.

Uses

1. Stage II–IV pressure ulcers
2. lower extremity ulcers
3. surgical wounds
4. infected wounds
5. diabetic ulcers

Caution

A gel will not form in a dry wound.

Examples

- AlgiDERM® (Bard)
- Kaltostat® (ConvaTec)
- Sorbsan (Bertek)
- Hyperion® (Hyperion Medical)
- Restore CalciCare Calcium Alginate Dressing (Hollister, Inc.)
- Kalginate (DeRoyal)
- Carasorb (Kendall)
- Ferris PolyMem Calcium Alginate Dressing (Ferris Mfg. Corp.)

TIPS
- Alginates are available in many configurations and sizes, making them practical for a multitude of wounds that require packing.
- Alginates may be flushed from the wound with normal saline.
- They can often be useful to decrease the frequency of dressing changes—most can remain in the wound until drainage is seen on the outer dressing.
- They are useful under compression wraps.

ANTIMICROBIALS

Antimicrobials can come as creams, ointments, impregnated gauzes, or other types of dressings.

Purpose

1. to control/reduce the number of microorganisms in a wound without damaging healthy tissue
2. to maintain a moist healing environment

Absorbency

1. depending upon the dressing, low to high
2. can require a secondary dressing

Uses

1. Stage II–IV pressure ulcers
2. lower extremity ulcers
3. surgical wounds

4. skin tears
5. grafts
6. infected wounds

Cautions

1. Read the manufacturer's recommendations.
2. Precautions must be taken when using iodine-based antimicrobials if there is a risk that the patient has a thyroid disorder.
3. These products are not intended to treat systemic infection.

Examples

- Thermazene Cream ("Silvadene") (Kendall)
- Iodoflex™ (Healthpoint)
- Iodosorb® (Healthpoint)
- Arglaes (Medline Industries, Inc.)
- Acticoat 7 (Smith & Nephew, Inc.)
- Acticoat Absorbent Dressing (Smith & Nephew, Inc.)
- Actisorb (Johnson & Johnson Medical)
- Kerlex AMD (Kendall)
- SilvaSorb Antimicrobial Silver Dressing (Medline Industries, Inc.)
- Silverlon Wound Pad Dressing (Argentum Medical LLC)
- Aquacel®Ag (ConvaTec)

FOAMS

Foam dressings are nonlinting and absorbent. Foams create a moist environment and provide thermal insulation to the wound. They are manufactured as pads, sheets, and pillow (cavity) dressings. They are generally nonadherent, may repel contaminants, are easy to apply and remove, absorb light to heavy amounts of exudate, and may be used under compression. They can be layered in combination with other materials. They also can have an adhesive border or a transparent film coating.

Purpose

1. absorb exudate
2. promote moist healing environment
3. insulation

Absorbency

Foams have high absorbency.

Uses

1. Stage II–IV pressure ulcers
2. lower extremity ulcers
3. skin tears

Cautions

1. Do not use on dry wounds.
2. Do not use with infected wounds.
3. Do not use as packing unless the product is specifically designed and labeled for packing, such as pillow "cavity" dressings.
4. Exudate may be released from foam if pressure occurs, causing maceration.

Examples

- Allevyn (Smith & Nephew, Inc.)
- PolyMem® (Ferris Mfg. Corp.)
- Cutinova® Foam (Beiersdorf-Jobst)
- Flexzan® (Bertek)
- Lyofoam® (ConvaTec)
- 3M Foam Dressing–Adhesive or Nonadhesive (3M Health Care)
- Biatain Foam Dressing (Coloplast)
- Tielle Hydropolymer Adhesive and Borderless Nonadhesive (Johnson & Johnson Medical)
- Mepilex–Borfer and Soft Silicone Absorbent Foam Dressing (Mölnlycke Health Care)
- Polyderm–Plus and Border (DeRoyal)

 TIPS
- Foams are easy to use and easy to teach patients/caregivers to use.
- Most are nonadherent, and they are available in many sizes and configurations.
- They are useful in decreasing the frequency of dressing changes, and most can be left in place until approximately 75% saturated.

HYDROCOLLOIDS

These are occlusive or semiocclusive dressings composed of materials such as gelatin, pectin, and/or carboxymethylcellulose. They generally provide a moist healing environment that allows clean wounds to granulate and necrotic wounds to debride autolytically. They are generally impermeable to bacteria and other contaminants. They are permeable to moisture vapor but not water. Hydrocolloids may be left in place for 3 to 5 days and may be used under compression. Absorbency depends upon composition. These dressings are self-adhering and available with and without a border. They contour easily.

Purpose

1. autolytic debridement
2. maintenance of moist healing environment
3. protection of the wound from external contaminants

Absorbency

1. low to moderate
2. may be enhanced with use of hydrocolloid paste

Uses

1. Stage I–III pressure ulcers
2. venous stasis ulcers

Cautions

1. Do not use on arterial or neuropathic ulcers.
2. Do not use if there is fragile skin surrounding the wound.
3. Do not use on infected wounds.

Examples

- DuoDERM® CGF® (ConvaTec)
- Restore™ (Hollister, Inc.)
- Comfeel® (Coloplast)
- OriDerm (Orion Medical Products)
- 3M Tegasorb™ (3M Health Care)
- Exuderm (Medline Industries, Inc.)
- NuDerm (Johnson & Johnson Medical)

TIPS
- Always use a larger size than the size of the wound; at least a 1-inch margin of hydrocolloid is needed. In difficult areas, up to a 3-inch margin may be needed for good adherence.
- You may need to create a picture frame with paper tape or transparent film.
- Many varieties are available in thin, conformable styles, often contoured to fit surface areas.
- Hydrocolloids may be useful under Montgomery straps to protect skin from adhesive.
- If used on "cratered" wounds, dead space must be filled in with hydrocolloid paste or alginate.

HYDROFIBERS

Hydrofibers are sterile nonwoven pads or ribbons composed of sodium carboxymethylcellulose fibers. They are conformable and absorbent, and they interact with wound exudate to form a gel. There must be enough exudate in the wound to convert the hydrofiber into a gel.

Purpose

1. packing
2. absorption
3. maintenance of a moist environment
4. autolytic debridement

Absorbency

Hydrofibers have high absorbency.

Uses

1. Stage II–IV pressure ulcers
2. lower extremity ulcers
3. surgical wounds

Cautions

1. Do not use on dry wounds.
2. Do not use on infected wounds.

Example

Aquacel™ Hydrofiber™ (ConvaTec)

TIPS
- Select a size that is at least an inch larger than the wound.
- If packing, do so lightly, do not overfill, and do not apply with pressure.
- Hydrofibers may be left in place for several days depending on the amount of exudate. If it does not become a gel-like sheet, flush it out with saline and consider using a less absorbent product.

HYDROGELS

Hydrogels are polymers, water- or glycerin-based amorphous gels, impregnated gauzes, or sheet dressings. They do not absorb large amounts of exudate because of their high water content. They help maintain a moist wound environment and promote granulation and epithelialization. Most dressings are soothing, reduce pain, rehydrate the wound bed, fill in dead spaces (impregnated gauze), and are easy to apply and remove. They generally require a secondary dressing.

Purpose

1. autolytic debridement
2. maintenance of a moist healing environment
3. hydration of dry wounds

Absorbency

Hydrogels have low absorbency.

Uses

1. Stage II–IV pressure ulcers
2. lower extremity ulcers
3. skin tears (in particular, sheet-style hydrogels)
4. surgical wounds

Caution

Do not use on heavily exudating wounds.

Examples

- Biolex™ (Bard)
- Carrasyn® (Carrington Laboratories, Inc.)
- Curasol® (Healthpoint)
- IntraSite (Smith & Nephew, Inc.)
- SoloSite® (Smith & Nephew, Inc.)
- Vigilon® (Bard)
- Restore Hydrogel Dressing (Hollister, Inc.)
- RadiGel (Carrington Laboratories, Inc.)
- Curafil Hydrogel Impregnated Gauze (Kendall)
- Curafil Gel Wound Dressing (Kendall)

 TIPS
- Hydrogels are available in sheets, impregnated gauze, and amorphous gel. Select the most appropriate form for the type and location of the wound.
- They may be refrigerated to enhance the soothing, pain-relieving property of the dressing.

TRANSPARENT FILMS

These adhesive, semipermeable, polyurethane membrane dressings vary in size and configuration. They are waterproof and are impermeable to contaminants and bacteria. However, they permit water vapor and atmospheric gases to cross the barrier. They do not absorb drainage. They retain moisture and are to be changed when fluid accumulates beneath them. Because these dressings are clear, wounds can be assessed without removing the dressing. They are available in a wide variety of sizes.

Purpose

1. encourages autolytic debridement
2. promotes moist healing environment
3. protects from external contaminants

Absorbency

Transparent films have low absorbency.

Uses

1. Stage I–II pressure ulcers
2. partial-thickness wounds
3. grafts
4. secondary, securing dressing over many other wound coverings

Cautions

1. Do not use on fragile skin surfaces.
2. Do not use on infected wounds.
3. Avoid using on wounds with large amounts of exudate.

Examples

- Tegaderm™ (3M Health Care)
- Bioclusive™ (Johnson & Johnson Medical)
- OpSite (Smith & Nephew, Inc.)
- DermaSite™ (Derma Sciences)
- Comfeel Film (Coloplast)
- Polyskin II Transparent Dressing (Kendall)
- BlisterFilm Transparent Dressing (Kendall)

TIPS • It is normal for exudate to be present on the wound surface under a film dressing. If the drainage is on the intact skin surrounding the wound, the dressing should be changed.
• If excessive exudate is on the wound surface, a tuberculin syringe may be used to aspirate the drainage. The puncture site can then be patched.

ENZYMATIC DEBRIDERS

By digesting necrotic tissue, these ointments debride wounds. Different types of enzymatic agents include proteolytic enzymes, fibrinolytic enzymes, collagenase, and papain. Their actions are specific to necrotic tissue. Most manufacturers report that they do not damage healthy tissue. (See Appendix 5–B.)

Purpose

1. debridement of necrotic tissue without damaging healthy tissue
2. maintenance of moist healing environment

Absorbency

1. low
2. secondary dressing (usually gauze moistened with saline) always required

Use

• necrotic wounds
• slough
• eschar

Caution

Do not use on fully granular wounds. Enzymatic debriders will not harm granulation tissue, but they are no longer necessary when all necrotic tissue is removed.

Example

• Collagenase Santyl® (Healthpoint). See Appendix 5–B. at the end of this chapter for step-by-step instructions for using Santyl.

GROWTH FACTORS

Growth factors are proteins that occur naturally in the human body. They cause cellular growth and cell migration and may regulate the wound healing process. They can be obtained through a process utilizing the body's platelets and macrophages, autologously derived, or made chemically or biochemically outside of the body, recombinant. Use of a growth factor is an adjunct to standard wound practice, such as debridement, pain relief, and infection control.

Purpose

1. cell proliferation
2. acceleration of healing

Absorbency

1. low
2. covered with moist gauze dressing

Use

Use growth factors for clean, granulating wounds only.

Cautions

1. Do not use on necrotic wounds.
2. Do not use on cancer sites or with patients with any neoplasms.
3. Store at reduced temperatures.

Example

Regranex® (Ortho-McNeil Pharmaceutical) (See **Exhibit 5–2**.)

 TIPS
- Growth factors are not effective on necrotic tissue.
- They are available by prescription only.
- Close adherence to manufacturer's instructions is imperative.

BIOSYNTHETICS

These may be gels or semiocclusive sheets derived from a natural source and may require freezing. They are used primarily on burn wounds and have also been found effective on a variety of skin-loss wounds, including skin tears and donor sites. They act as a skin substitute. They foster healing by reepithelialization. They may be nonadherent. The product is surgically applied to the wound surface by a wound care practitioner and covered with a dressing.

Exhibit 5–2 Patient Guide: Regranex®

USING REGRANEX® GEL THE PROPER WAY, EVERY DAY

1. Wash hands thoroughly before applying Regranex® Gel.
2. Before you apply Regranex® Gel, remove the dressing from the wound and rinse the wound gently with saline solution or water.
3. Do not touch the tip of the tube to any surface. Use an application aid such as a cotton swab or tongue depressor.
4. Apply a carefully measured quantity of Regranex® Gel to the wound (enough to cover the surface) as instructed by your health care professional. Do not apply a thick layer—it will not increase the effect of Regranex® Gel.
5. After applying Regranex® Gel, dress the wound as instructed by your doctor or health care professional.
   - Place a suitable size, saline-moistened pad over the wound. The correct size pad should cover the wound completely and have at least an inch to spare all around. Do not try to trim the pad after applying it to the wound.
   - Wrap a gauze bandage snugly over the pad and secure it with adhesive tape. Make sure that the adhesive side of the tape is secured onto the gauze and not to your skin.
   - Only plain gauze should be used. Any dressings containing ointments or other ingredients should be avoided.
   - After bandaging, check to make sure that the bandage is secure enough so that it doesn't slip off, but not so tight as to be uncomfortable or hinder your circulation.

OTHER INSTRUCTIONS

- You should use a mirror to check both of your feet every day. Adjust the mirror at different angles to get the best view of your feet.
- Other wound care products have not been studied for use with Regranex® Gel. Therefore, when using Regranex® Gel, avoid other creams, gels, or ointments at the site of the wound.
- After 12 hours, remove the dressing and gently rinse the wound with saline solution or water. DO NOT APPLY ANY REGRANEX® GEL AT THIS TIME. Apply a new moist dressing on the wound.
- Continue to use Regranex® Gel until your wound has completely healed or until your health care professional tells you to stop.
- Visit your health care professional regularly during the course of treatment.
- If you feel any discomfort, or have any questions, contact your health care professional immediately.
- Regranex® Gel must be stored in the refrigerator at all times. DO NOT FREEZE.

QUESTIONS & ANSWERS

Q. **What is Regranex® Gel, and what does it do for diabetic foot ulcers?**

A. Regranex® Gel is a prescription drug for the treatment of diabetic foot ulcers. It contains a factor normally found in the blood (referred to as a platelet-derived growth factor), which is part of the body's natural healing process. Some wounds take a long time to heal, and others may not heal at all. Regranex® Gel can help this problem in many patients by delivering the growth factor directly to the ulcer in a simple-to-use gel.

Q. **How is Regranex® Gel different from other wound care therapies?**

A. You may have heard of, or even tried, other treatments for diabetic foot ulcers. Most of these treatments only help keep the wound clean and moist. Regranex® Gel is different because it is clinically proven to help heal more wounds.

Q. **What, if any, side effects can I expect from using Regranex® Gel?**

A. When used correctly, Regranex® Gel is well tolerated. A small percentage of patients treated with Regranex® Gel experienced local irritation or rash. If you experience any such effect, you should discuss it with your doctor or health care professional.

Source: Courtesy of Ortho-McNeil Pharmaceutical, (2000). Raritan, NJ.

Exhibit 5–3 Nuggets from Experience

MACERATION

Maceration is softening of tissue due to excessive moisture. Wound edges become white and soft. When maceration occurs around wound edges, skin barrier cream or wipes should be applied. If maceration continues to occur, consider a more absorptive dressing or increase the frequency of dressing changes until drainage decreases.

HYPERGRANULATION

When granulation tissue proliferates and overlaps the wound bed, epithelialization cannot occur. Consider a more absorptive dressing to manage the hypergranulation tissue. If this is not effective, paint the tissue daily with betadine to suppress the hypergranulation and allow the epithelial cells to migrate over the granulation tissue. Discontinue the betadine when the hypergranulation tissue is resolved. Silver nitrate can be used to cauterize the hypergranulation tissue and allow epithelialization to occur. Repeat applications may be necessary (**Figure 5–2**; Color Plate 8).

SHARPS DEBRIDEMENT

When bleeding occurs after sharps debridement, appropriate care is a clean, dry dressing for 8 to 24 hours. Then resume moist wound care.

MALIGNANCY

Be aware that unusual chronic wounds and wounds that fail to heal after adequate therapy may require a biopsy to rule out malignancy.

ROLLED EDGES

Full-thickness chronic wounds may have thick, rolled edges. Epithelial cells have migrated down and around the wound edges. For the wound to complete the healing process, silver nitrate can be applied to the wound edges. Another choice is to allow the wound edges to become macerated. The goal is to break down the rolled edges so that epithelialization of the wound surface can occur.

HEEL ULCERS WITH DRY ESCHAR

The *Agency for Health Care Policy and Research Guidelines* state that "heel ulcers with dry eschar need not be debrided if they do not have edema, erythema, fluctuance, or drainage. Assess these wounds daily to monitor for pressure ulcer complications" (Bergstrom et al., 1994, p. 49).

OCCLUSIVE DRESSINGS

Do not use occlusive dressings such as hydrocolloids on infected wounds or wounds with potential for anaerobic infection. Do not use on deep cavity wounds or wounds with undermining or sinus tracts. Discontinue the dressing if undermining or sinus tracts develop.

DRY GANGRENE

Do not attempt wound care of dry gangrene. If the physician is aware of the situation and a conservative course of treatment is indicated, keep the site clean, dry, and protected. Monitor for worsening condition.

NECROTIC TISSUE ON ISCHEMIC LIMBS

If ischemia is present, monitor wounds for signs and symptoms of worsening condition. If the wound is eschar-covered without signs of infection, keep the site clean, dry, and protected. If the wound is open, wound gel may be used. The wound will not heal without an adequate blood supply, but not all patients are candidates for surgery. Remember that aggressive wound care may, in fact, hasten the time of amputation.

WOUNDS/PRESSURE ULCERS ON PATIENTS AT THE END OF THEIR LIFE

Choose a dressing that is an appropriate treatment for the wound, that will be comfortable for the patient, and that reduces the frequency of dressing changes. For a heavily exudating wound, a hydrofiber or calcium alginate dressing would absorb drainage, keep the patient comfortable, and reduce the frequency of dressing changes. If the wound is dry, a gel would keep the wound moist, be comfortable, and protect the wound. A specialty mattress for pressure reduction or pressure relief could prevent further breakdown and be comfortable for the patient.

Source: Adapted from Agency for Healthcare Policy and Research. (1994). *AHCPR Treatment Guidelines #15.* Rockville, MD: U.S. Department of Health and Human Services.

Examples

- Biobrane® (Bertek)
- BGC Matrix® (Brennen Medical Inc.)
- Inerpan® (Kendall)
- Apligraf® (Novartis)
- Integra™ (Integra LifeSciences Corporation)

COLLAGEN

Collagen is a fibrous, insoluble protein produced by fibroblasts and derived from bovine hide. Collagen dressings may stimulate new tissue development and wound debridement. Collagen dressings may encourage the deposition and organization of newly formed collagen fibers and granulation tissue in the wound bed. The dressings absorb exudate and maintain a moist wound-healing environment. The dressing can be 100% collagen or combined with other products such as alginates. They are nonadherent and are easy to apply and remove.

Figure 5–2 Local Wound Managment Interventions Algorithm.
Source: Courtesy of Bonnie Sure Ralstad, RN, BA, CWOCN. Copyright © 2000.

Examples

- Fibracol™ (Johnson & Johnson Medical)
- Cellerete Rx (Hymed Group Corp.)
- Promogran Matrix Wound Dressing (Johnson & Johnson Medical)

Caution

Do not use on dry wounds or with patients sensitive to bovine products.

RELATED WOUND TREATMENTS

Negative Pressure Wound Therapy (NPWT)

NPWT is also known as Topical Negative Pressure Therapy. This is a system that uses controlled negative pressure (vacuum) to help promote wound healing.

Clinical benefits of Negative Pressure Wound Therapy can include:

- decreased edema of periwound area
- increased local vascularity
- decreased bacterial load
- increased rate of granulation tissue formation
- promotion of epithelialization
- maintenance of moist wound environment
- increased rate of wound contraction
- accurate measurement of wound drainage

Indications:

- dehisced surgical wounds
- complex operative wounds left open to heal by secondary intention
- diabetic ulcers
- chronic wounds
- traumatic wounds
- acute wounds
- venous or arterial ulcers that do not respond to standard therapy
- pressure ulcers
- flaps and grafts
- partial and full thickness burns
- chronic or acute enteric fistulas

Contraindications:

- malignancy
- untreated osteomyelitis

- fistulas to organs or body cavities
- necrotic tissue with eschar present
- exposed arteries, veins or organs
- uncontrolled pain

Precautions should be taken with patients exhibiting:

- active bleeding
- difficult hemostasis
- anticoagulant therapy

When placing a NPWT dressing in proximity to blood vessels, the clinician should take care to ensure that all vessels are adequately protected with overlying fascia, tissue, or other protective barriers. Greater care should be taken with respect to weakened, irradiated, or sutured blood vessels. Follow universal precautions.

Some NPWT systems are foam based (Wound VAC and Svedman Wound Treatment System). The Engenex System is a Bio-Dome Technology. All remaining systems are gauze based. Each kind of system is marketed as NPWT.

Wound site should be inspected for signs of infection with each dressing change. Any changes should be reported to the physician. The patient can have NPWT therapy started at the hospital, extended care, or home. If started at the hospital, the NPWT therapy can be transitioned home or to an extended care facility.

Hyperbaric Oxygen (HBO)

Hyperbaric oxygen therapy is inhalation of 100% oxygen delivered at pressures of more than 1 atmosphere (ATA). Hyperbaric oxygen is provided in enclosed chambers in individual (monoplace) and group (multiplace) settings. It is believed to promote wound healing by stimulating fibroblast, collagen synthesis, epithelialization, and controlling infection.

Indications

The American Diabetic Association indicates that adjunctive HBO may be reasonable to use in treating severe limb- or life-threatening wounds that have not responded to other treatments. Other wounds that respond to HBO are those that have been acutely or chronically compromised by hypoxia and/or infection. Clinical conditions associated with these types of wounds are peripheral vascular disease, diabetes, radiation necrosis, mixed soft tissue infections, refractory osteomyelitis, and selected traumatic wounds. HBO may be considered in combination with good wound care when traditional wound treatment plans have failed.

COMPOSITES

A composite is a combination of two or more physically distinct products manufactured as a single dressing that provides multiple functions.

Examples

- Covaderm Plus® (DeRoyal Wound Care)
- Alldress® Absorbent Film Dressing (Mölnlycke)
- Visasorb Wound Dressing (Kendall)
- CovRSite Plus Composite Dressing (Smith & Nephew, Inc.)
- Repel Wound Dressing (MPM Medical Sciences, Inc.)

COMPRESSION WRAPS

Compression wraps help to heal venous ulcers by reducing dependent edema and facilitating venous return through the enhancement of the effects of the foot and calf muscle pumps. They are available as single or multiple layers and elastic stockings.

Examples

- Profore Four Layer Bandaging System (Smith & Nephew, Inc.)
- Unna-flex® Elastic Unna Boot (ConvaTec)
- CircAid® (Coloplast)
- Jobst® UlcerCare (Beiersdorf-Jobst, Inc.)
- Dyna-flex™ Multi-Layer Compression System (Johnson & Johnson Medical)

Caution

Compression wraps are contraindicated with arterial disease.

REFERENCES

Bergstrom, N., et al. (1994). *Treatment of pressure ulcers*. Clinical Practice Guideline No. 15. AHCPR Publication No. 95-0652. Rockville, MD: U.S. Department of Health and Human Services. Public Health Services, Agency for Health Care Policy and Research.

Boykin, J. V. (2001). Treatment options and questions and answers about hyperbaric oxygen therapy. *Advances in Skin and Wound Care, 14*(5), 232–234.

Mendez-Eastman, S. (2001). Guidelines for using negative pressure wound therapy. *Advances in Skin and Wound Care, 14*(6), 314–325.

BIBLIOGRAPHY

Baranoski, S. (1999). Wound dressings: Challenging decisions. *Home Healthcare Nurse, 17*(1), 19–25.

Baranoski, S., & Ayello, E. A. (2004). Wound treatment options. In S. Baranoski & E. A. Ayello (Eds.), *Wound care essentials: Practice principles* (pp. 127–156). Philadelphia: Lippincott Williams & Wilkins.

Houghton, P., & Campbell, K. (1999). Choosing an adjunctive therapy for the treatment of chronic wounds. *Ostomy/Wound Management, 45*(8), 43–52.

Long, M. A., & Blevins, A. (2009, March/April). Options in negative pressure wound therapy. *Journal of Wound, Ostomy, and Continence Nursing, 36*(2), 202–211.

Moues, C. M. (2009, March). Five millennia of wound care products—What is new? A literature review. *Ostomy/Wound Management, 55*(3), 16–30.

Rolstad, B. S., & Ovington, L. G., (2007). Principles of wound management. In R. Bryant & D. Nix (Eds.), *Acute and chronic wounds: Current management concepts* (3rd ed., pp. 391–426). St. Louis, MO: Mosby.

Sibbald, R. (1998). An approach to leg and foot ulcers: A brief overview. *Ostomy/Wound Management, 44*(9), 28–35.

Sprung, P., et al. (1998). Hydrogels and hydrocolloids: An objective products comparison. *Ostomy/Wound Management, 44*(1), 36–53.

Sussman, C., & Bates-Jensen, B. (1998). *Wound care: A collaborative practice manual for physical therapists and nurses.* Gaithersburg, MD: Aspen.

Wound Ostomy and Continence Nurses Society. (2003). *Guideline for prevention and management of pressure ulcers.* WOCN Clinical Practice Guideline, No. 2. Glenview IL: Author.

Resources/Manufacturers' List

Manufacturer	Phone	Website
3M Health Care	1-800-228-3957	www.3M.com/healthcare
Bard Medical Division	1-800-526-4455	www.bardmedical.com
Beiersdorf-Jobst, Inc.	1-800-537-1063	www.beiersdorf.com
BioCore Medical Technologies, Inc.	1-888-565-5243	www.biocore.com
Blue Sky Medical	1-877-7BlueSky	www.blueskymedical.com
Brennen Medical Inc.	1-800-328-9105	www.brennenmed.com/
Carrington Labs	1-800-527-5216	www.carringtonlabs.com
Coloplast	1-800-533-0464	www.coloplast.com
ConvaTec	1-800-422-8811	www.convatec.com
Derma Sciences, Inc.	1-800-825-4325	www.dermasciences.com
DeRoyal Wound Care	1-800-337-6925	www.deroyal.com
Healthpoint	1-800-441-8227	www.healthpoint.com
Hollister, Inc.	1-800-323-4060	www.hollister.com
Johnson & Johnson Medical Division of Ethicon, Inc.	1-800-255-2500	www.jnj.com
Kendall Health Care Products, Inc.	1-800-962-9888	www.kendallhq.com
Medline Industries, Inc.	1-800-633-5463	www.medline.net
Mölnlycke	1-800-659-8037	www.molnlycke.com
Novartis	1-888-432-5232	www.apligraf.com
Ortho-McNeil Pharmaceutical Inc.	1-888-734-7263	www.regranex.com
Smith & Nephew, Inc.	1-800-876-1261	www.npwt.com

Patient Guide: Santyl

SANTYL®

Caring for the Skin Ulcer

These instructions are general; be sure to follow your healthcare professional's directions for your specific-condition.

Change the dressing on the skin ulcer at least once every day. If the area becomes soiled or damp, change the dressing as often as needed, and follow all of the steps listed here.

A healthcare professional may need to cut through some of the dead tissue in the skin ulcer and remove as much of it as possible. This should not be painful. DO NOT try to do this yourself.

1. Wash your hands with soap and water. Dry with a clean towel.

2. Gently clean the open wound according to instructions specified by your healthcare professional.

3. Rinse the wound with normal saline solution (your healthcare professional can tell you how to obtain or make this) to remove any dead skin.

4. If you have been instructed to use an antibiotic powder on the area, sprinkle a light dusting of powder onto the wound area.

5. Apply Santyl® ointment:
   a. For a shallow wound, put Santyl® ointment on a sterile gauze pad and then apply it directly to the wound, so that the ointment touches the ulcer surface. Do not get the ointment on the surrounding skin.
   b. For a deep ulcer, use a clean wooden tongue depressor to gently apply Santyl® ointment to the wound surface. Do not get the ointment on the surrounding skin. Throw the tongue depressor away with the soiled dressing in a closed plastic bag.

6. Cover the wound with a dry, sterile gauze pad. Secure the pad with nonallergenic paper tape. Use as little tape as possible to keep the dressing in place. Leave the sides of the gauze pad open.

1. The skin ulcer is filled with dead skin.

2. Antibiotic fights infection and Santyl® ointment removes dead skin.

3. Healthy pink cells start to form around the edge and on the surface. Discontinue Santyl® when granulation tissue is well established.

4. Healthy skin tissue fills in the wound.

Is Your Ulcer Getting Better?

A skin ulcer can be like an iceberg: There may be a large area below the surface of the ulcer that is not easily seen. For healing to take place below the surface, the dead skin on the top has to be removed first. That's part of the job of Santyl® ointment—to clear away the dead tissue cells.

When Santyl® ointment is used properly, the wound might get bigger at first. This is actually a good sign. So is an unpleasant odor—it means the wound is draining and getting cleaner, and that's a positive step in the healing process.

As the dead tissue disappears, healthy pink skin cells will start to form around the edges of the wound. With time and proper care, healthy tissue will fill in the wound.

The Healing Process Over Time

1. The skin ulcer is filled with dead skin.
2. Antibiotic fights infection and Santyl® ointment removes dead skin.
3. Healthy pink cells start to form around the edge and on the surface. Santyl® ointment can be used, as per the package insert (PDR), until granulation tissue is well established.
4. Healthy skin tissue fills in the wound.

Wound Types Commonly Seen by Healthcare Professionals

Pressure Ulcers

Donna Oddo

Pressure ulcers, also commonly called decubitus ulcers, are areas where pressure has destroyed soft tissue. Typically located over bony prominences, pressure ulcers may occur in any area where pressure can adversely affect the soft tissue.

Assess all patients for their risk of skin breakdown upon admission and periodically throughout their length of care. Once a pressure ulcer develops, the patient is subject to increased pain and possible infection. This can lead to loss of function or loss of the limb, as well as fluid imbalances, malnourishment, and disfigurement. Patients may then require long-term nursing intervention and/or surgical intervention.

Prevention is imperative. Prevention measures should focus on reducing the pressure, maintaining and improving the patient's tissue tolerance to pressure, and educating the patient and caregiver.

However, Kennedy Terminal Ulcers have been identified as ulcers occurring at the end of life. They are caused by poor vascular circulation. It is important to determine the etiology of a wound on the sacrococcygeal area. If the wound appears as a discoloration of the skin in the shape of a butterfly or pear; has a sudden onset; or is purple red, blue, or black with irregular borders, it may be a Kennedy Terminal Ulcer. The body's vascular system is no longer able to profuse the skin. This is a consequence of the dying process, and death usually occurs within hours to days. Palliative care should be provided. See the article, "Pressure or Pathology," listed in the bibliography of this chapter.

ETIOLOGY

In normal tissue, a balance exists between interstitial and solid tissue pressure. Outside pressure forces can lead to

- an increase in interstitial fluid pressure
- a rise in arteriolar and capillary pressure
- filtering of a fluid from capillaries, resulting in
  - edema
  - autolysis

- occlusion of lymph vessels
- accumulation of anaerobic waste
- necrosis

Approximately 70% of the tissue damage occurs below the skin surface.

ASSESSMENT

When staging a pressure ulcer (**Exhibit 6–1**), remember:

- Stage the wound according to the depth of tissue damage visible.
- If damaged tissue is not visible, the wound cannot be staged. Necrotic tissue must be removed before damage can be assessed. (**Figure 6–1**; **Color Plate 9**.)

Exhibit 6–1 Pressure Ulcer Stages Revised by NPUAP

February 2007—The National Pressure Ulcer Advisory Panel has redefined the definition of a pressure ulcer and the stages of pressure ulcers, including the original four stages and adding two stages on deep tissue injury and unstageable pressure ulcers. This work is the culmination of over 5 years of work beginning with the identification of deep tissue injury in 2001.

Pressure Ulcer Definition

A pressure ulcer is localized injury to the skin and/or underlying tissue usually over a bony prominence, as a result of pressure, or pressure in combination with shear and/or friction. A number of contributing or confounding factors are also associated with pressure ulcers; the significance of these factors is yet to be elucidated.

Pressure Ulcer Stages

Suspected Deep Tissue Injury: A purple or maroon localized area of discolored intact skin or a blood-filled blister due to damage of underlying soft tissue from pressure and/or shear may indicate deep tissue injury. The area may be preceded by tissue that is painful, firm, mushy, boggy, warmer, or cooler as compared to adjacent tissue.

Further description: Deep tissue injury may be difficult to detect in individuals with dark skin tones. Its evolution may include a thin blister over a dark wound bed. The wound may further evolve and become covered by thin eschar. The evolution may be rapid, exposing additional layers of tissue even with optimal treatment. (**Figure 6–2**; **Color plate 27**)

Stage I: Stage I is intact skin with nonblanchable redness of a localized area, usually over a bony prominence. Darkly pigmented skin may not have visible blanching; its color may differ from the surrounding area. (**Figure 6–3**; **Color plate 10**)

Further description: The area may be painful, firm, soft, warmer, or cooler as compared to adjacent tissue. Stage I may be difficult to detect in individuals with dark skin tones and may indicate "at risk" persons (a heralding sign of risk).

Stage II: Stage II is a partial thickness loss of dermis presenting as a shallow open ulcer with a red-pink wound bed, without slough. It may also present as an intact or open/ruptured serum-filled blister.

Further description: Stage II presents as a shiny or dry shallow ulcer without slough or bruising.* This stage should not be used to describe skin tears, tape burns, perineal dermatitis, maceration, or excoriation. (**Figure 6–4**; **Color plate 11**)

Stage III: Stage III is a full thickness tissue loss. Subcutaneous fat may be visible, but bone, tendon, or muscle is not exposed. Slough may be present but does not obscure the depth of tissue loss. It may include undermining and tunneling. (**Figure 6–5**; **Color plate 12**)

Further description: The depth of a Stage III pressure ulcer varies by anatomical location. The bridge of the nose, ear, occiput, and malleolus do not have subcutaneous tissue, and Stage III ulcers can be shallow. In contrast, areas of significant adiposity can develop extremely deep Stage III pressure ulcers. Bone/tendon is not visible or directly palpable.

Stage IV: Stage IV is a full thickness tissue loss with exposed bone, tendon, or muscle. Slough or eschar may be present on some parts of the wound bed. It often includes undermining and tunneling. (**Figure 6–6**; **Color plate 13**)

Further description: The depth of a Stage IV pressure ulcer varies by anatomical location. The bridge of the nose, ear, occiput, and malleolus do not have subcutaneous tissue, and these ulcers can be shallow. Stage IV ulcers can extend into muscle and/or supporting structures (e.g., fascia, tendon, or joint capsule) making osteomyelitis possible. Exposed bone/tendon is visible or directly palpable.

Unstageable: Full thickness tissue loss in which the base of the ulcer is covered by slough (yellow, tan, gray, green, or brown) and/or eschar (tan, brown, or black) in the wound bed.

Further description: Until enough slough and/or eschar is removed to expose the base of the wound, the true depth, and therefore stage, cannot be determined. Stable (dry, adherent, intact without erythema or fluctuance) eschar on the heels serves as "the body's natural (biological) cover" and should not be removed.

The staging system was defined by Shea in 1975 and provides a name to the amount of anatomical tissue loss. The original definitions were confusing to many clinicians and lead to inaccurate staging of ulcers associated or due to perineal dermatitis and those due to deep tissue injury.

The proposed definitions were refined by the NPUAP with input from an on-line evaluation of their face validity, accuracy clarity, succinctness, utility, and discrimination. This process was completed online and provided input to the Panel for continued work. The proposed final definitions were reviewed by a consensus conference and their comments were used to create the final definitions. "NPUAP is pleased to have completed this important task and looks forward to the inclusion of these definitions into practice, education and research," said Joyce Black, NPUAP President and Chairperson of the Staging Task Force.

For more information, contact npuap.org or 202-521-6789

Source: Courtesy of National Pressure Ulcer Advisory Panel, (2007). Washington, DC.

*Bruising indicates suspected deep tissue injury.

Figure 6–1 Pressure Ulcer on Sacrum. Unable to stage due to yellow necrotic tissue in the base of the wound.

Clinical Objectives:

(1) Clean

(2) Remove slough

(3) Manage exudate

(4) Keep moist

(5) Protect from incontinence

(6) Relieve pressure

See Color Plate 9.

Figure 6–2 Suspected deep tissue injury on a person with dark skin.

See Color Plate 27.

Figure 6–3 Stage I Pressure Ulcer. Nonblanchable erythema.

Clinical Objectives:
(1) Keep clean
(2) Cover and protect
(3) Eliminate pressure, friction, and shear
See Color Plate 10.

Figure 6–4 Stage II Pressure Ulcer at Sacral Region. Thin layer of desiccated tissue.

Clinical Objectives:
(1) Clean
(2) Protect from incontinence
(3) Keep moist
(4) Prevent pressure, friction, and shear
See Color Plate 11.

Figure 6–5 Healing Stage III Pressure Ulcer.
Clinical Objectives:
(1) Cleanse
(2) Keep moist
See Color Plate 12.

(3) Manage exudate
(4) Relieve pressure, prevent friction and shear

yellow slough

black eschar

red
granulation
tissue

Figure 6–6 Stage IV Pressure Ulcer on Sacrum with Necrotic Tissue and Undermining.
Clinical Objectives:
(1) Remove devitalized tissue
    (slough and eschar)
(2) Clean
(3) Keep moist

(4) Manage exudate
(5) Protect from incontinence
(6) Relieve pressure, prevent friction and shear
See Color Plate 13.

> **TIP**
>
> **BRADEN SCALE: HELPFUL TIPS** When scoring each risk factor, if the assessment lies between two scores, use the lower score. When testing the patient's sensory perception, be sure to pinch the upper arm or thigh. Do not pinch fingers, hands, or nail beds. When testing the patient's sensory perception:
>
> - if reflex response only, score 1
> - if responds, but doesn't open eyes, score 3
> - no paralysis, score 4
>
> When testing the patient's activity:
>
> - walks to bathroom or chair only, score 3
>
> When testing mobility, do not consider the caregiver turning the patient.
>
> - severe depression or medicated, score 2
> - strongly prefers a position, score 3
>
> When testing the patient's nutrition:
>
> - usual intake—not temporary intake; e.g., NPO for test
>
> An excellent resource for prevention and treatment of pressure ulcers can be found in *Guideline for Prevention and Management of Pressure Ulcers*. Copyright 2002 by the Wound Ostomy and Continence Nurses Society. Refer to its Web site www.wocn.org, or call 888-224-WOCN.
>
> Additional pressure ulcer assessment information can be found at the National Pressure Ulcer Advisory Panel Web site, www.npuap.org, and at the Braden Scale Web site, www.bradenscale.com.

- It is inappropriate to backstage an ulcer as it heals. Stage is consistently kept at the deepest level of damage; e.g., Stage IV will always be a Stage IV. The wound may fill with granulation tissue and close but will never be considered a Stage I, II, or III at any point in the healing process.
- Staging can be difficult. If you are unsure of how to accurately stage a pressure ulcer then describe what you see. Consult information sources on wound assessment for instructions.

PREVENTION

Assessing Risk

To identify at-risk patients, use one scale consistently, such as the Braden Scale (**Exhibit 6–2**):

> **TIP**
>
> In home care, the scales broadly identify patients at risk. Be certain to assess factors in the home environment (e.g., caregiver ability and willingness, quality and amounts of oral intake, upkeep of patient's bedding and surroundings).

- on admission
- on recertification or reactivation to services
- when the condition of the patient changes

To complete the Braden Scale:

1. In the last column, write the number that most closely matches the patient's condition.
2. Total the column.

Exhibit 6–2 Braden Scale for Predicting Pressure Sore Risk

Patient's Name _____   Evaluator's Name _____   Date of Assessment _____

SENSORY PERCEPTION ability to respond meaningfully to pressure-related discomfort	1. Completely Limited: Unresponsive (does not moan, flinch, or gasp) to painful stimuli due to diminished level of consciousness or sedation. OR Limited ability to feel pain over most of body.	2. Very Limited: Responds only to painful stimuli. Cannot communicate discomfort except by moaning or restlessness. OR Has a sensory impairment that limits the ability to feel pain or discomfort over one-half of the body.	3. Slightly Limited: Responds to verbal commands but cannot always communicate discomfort or need to be turned. OR Has some sensory impairment that limits ability to feel pain or discomfort in one or two extremities.	4. No Impairment: Responds to verbal commands. Has no sensory deficit that would limit ability to feel or voice pain or discomfort.
MOISTURE degree to which skin is exposed to moisture	1. Constantly Moist: Skin is kept moist almost constantly by perspiration, urine, etc. Dampness is detected every time patient is moved or turned.	2. Very Moist: Skin is often, but not always, moist. Linen must be changed at least once a shift.	3. Occasionally Moist: Skin is occasionally moist, requiring an extra linen change approximately once a day.	4. Rarely Moist: Skin is usually dry, linen only requires changing at routine intervals.
ACTIVITY degree of physical activity	1. Bedfast: Confined to bed.	2. Chairfast: Ability to walk severely limited or nonexistent. Cannot bear own weight and/or must be assisted into chair or wheelchair.	3. Walks Occasionally: Walks occasionally during day but for very short distances, with or without assistance. Spends majority of each shift in bed or chair.	4. Walks Frequently: Walks outside the room at least twice a day and inside room at least every 2 hours during waking hours.
MOBILITY ability to change and control body position	1. Completely Immobile: Does not make even slight changes in body extremity position without assistance.	2. Very Limited: Makes occasional slight changes in body or extremity position but unable to make frequent or significant changes independently.	3. Slightly Limited: Makes frequent though slight changes in body or extremity positions independently.	4. No Limitations: Makes major and frequent changes in position without assistance.

	1. Very Poor:	2. Probably Inadequate:	3. Adequate:	4. Excellent:
NUTRITION usual food intake pattern	Never eats a complete meal. Rarely eats more than a third of any food offered. Eats two servings or less of protein (meat or dairy products) per day. Takes fluids poorly. Does not take a liquid dietary supplement. OR Is NPO and/or maintained on clear liquids or IVs for more than five days.	Rarely eats a complete meal and generally eats only about half of any food offered. Protein intake includes only three servings of meat or dairy products per day. Occasionally will take a dietary supplement. OR Receives less than optimum amount of liquid diet or tube feeding.	Eats over half of most meals. Eats a total of four servings of protein (meat, dairy products) each day. Occasionally will refuse a meal, but will usually take a supplement if offered. OR Is on a tube feeding or TPN regimen that probably meets most of nutritional needs.	Eats most of every meal. Never refuses a meal. Usually eats a total of four or more servings of meat and dairy products. Occasionally eats between meals. Does not require supplementation.
	1. Problem:	**2. Potential Problem:**	**3. No Apparent Problem:**	
FRICTION AND SHEAR	Requires moderate to maximum assistance in moving. Complete lifting without sliding against sheets is impossible. Frequently slides down in bed or chair, requiring frequent repositioning with maximum assistance. Spasticity, contractures, or agitation leads to almost constant friction.	Moves feebly or requires minimum assistance. During a move, skin probably slides to some extent against sheets, chair, restraints, or other devices. Maintains relatively good position in chair or bed most of the time but occasionally slides down.	Moves in bed and in chair independently and has sufficient muscle strength to lift up completely during move. Maintains good position in bed or chair at all times.	

Total Score _____

A total score of 15–18 or less is considered at risk; 13 or 14 is considered moderate risk; 10–12 is considered high risk; and 6–9 or below is considered very high risk.

Risk Factors

Extrinsic Risk Factors

- pressure
- immobility
- limited mobility
- moisture
- heat
- friction
- shear

Intrinsic Risk Factors

- poor nutritional status (refer to **Exhibit 6–3**, the Nutritional Risk Screening Form)

> **TIP** A good indicator of a patient's nutritional status is a serum prealbumin or albumin level.

- sensory deficit
- cardiopulmonary compromise
- anemia
- tissue fragility

The At-Risk Patient

Pressure Redistribution

Refer to Medicare Part B Guidelines for Specialty Mattresses in the Home (**Exhibit 6–4**). Group 1 support surfaces may be used for prevention.

- air or foam overlays
- nonpowered mattress replacements

Wheelchair cushions should be fitted by patient need and reassessed periodically for efficiency. Avoid use of donut-style seat cushions.

Patient Movement

- Reposition the at-risk patient every 2 hours while in bed. Ideally adjust the schedule to best meet the patient's needs.
- Limit sitting intervals to 2 hours, with weight shifts every 15 minutes.
- Perform range-of-motion exercises daily.
- Maintain good alignment.

Exhibit 6–3 Nutritional Risk Screening Form

Name: _____ Pt #: _____ DOB: _____

Physician's Name: _____ Phone #: _____

Diagnosis: _____ Diet Order: _____

Height: _____   Weight: Current _____   1 month ago _____   6 months ago _____

NUTRITION RISK INDICATORS

Check/date all that apply.

Indicator   **Criteria**

❏ Weight change from usual   ❏ > 10-lb change in 3 months   ❏ BMI < 22
                                ❏ 5% weight change in 1 month

❏ High-risk diagnosis   ❏ Hip fracture/replacement   ❏ Pneumonia
                                ❏ Pressure ulcer, wounds   ❏ Cancer
                                ❏ GI disease   ❏ CHF
                                ❏ Dysphagia   ❏ COPD
                                ❏ Other _____   ❏ Depression
                                                                  ❏ CVA
                                                                  ❏ Diabetes
                                                                  ❏ HIV/AIDS
                                                                  ❏ Renal failure

❏ Complex diet order   ❏ > 3 dietary modifications   ❏ Tube feeding
                                ❏ Receiving medical nutritional   ❏ Parenteral nutrition
                                   supplement   support
                                ❏ Transitioning from EN to oral,
                                   or PN to EN

❏ Physical signs   ❏ Poor skin turgor   ❏ Edema
                                ❏ Dry mucous membranes   ❏ Oral lesions
                                ❏ Muscle wasting   ❏ Dull, dry, and/or brittle
                                ❏ Weakness/tremors   hair
                                ❏ Psychosocial factors

❏ Psychosocial factors   ❏ No caregiver in the home   ❏ Limited mobility (inability
                                ❏ No transportation   to prepare food)
                                                                  ❏ Limited funds to buy food

(continues)

Exhibit 6–3 *continued*

❑ Other: _____

Signed: _____ Date: _____

NUTRITION RISK DETERMINATION

❑ Low risk (no indicators checked). Reassess in _____ days.
❑ Moderate risk (one indicator checked).
❑ High risk (two or more indicators checked).

INTERVENTIONS

❑ Initiate interdisciplinary care plan for _____
❑ Provide Ensure® Patient Starter Kit
❑ Request RD chart consult
❑ Request RD home referral

Signed: _____ Date: _____

Source: Courtesy of Ross Products Division of Abbott Laboratories, Inc., (1999), Columbus, OH.

- Use turn sheets and lifting devices.
- Use trapeze when indicated.
- Do not elevate the head of the bed over 30 degrees (may lead to shearing at sacrum).
- The heels should be floated off the bed surface at all times.

Nutrition

Nutritional assessment for the at-risk patient may include:

- albumin level
  - normal range 5 3.5–5 g/dl (grams per deciliter)
  - mild depletion 5 2.8–3.4 g/dl
  - moderate depletion 5 2.1–2.7 g/dl
  - severe depletion, 2.1 g/dl
- prealbumin
  - normal range 5 19–43 mg/dl
  - mild depletion 5 10–15 mg/dl

Exhibit 6–4 Medicare Part B Guidelines for Specialty Mattresses in the Home

Patient qualifications are expressed in summary terms. For clarification and specific terms, contact your DMERC. Guidelines are subject to change without any notice.

GROUP 1

These products are overlays and nonpowered replacements. Patients should have at least one of these characteristics:

- immobility
- a pressure ulcer on the trunk or pelvis
- limited mobility plus one of the following:
  - incontinence
  - malnutrition
  - altered sensory perception
  - compromised circulatory status

GROUP 2

These products are low-air-loss or alternating pressure mattress replacements. Patients should have at least one of these characteristics:

- large or multiple Stage III or IV pressure ulcer(s) on the trunk or pelvis
- multiple Stage II pressure ulcers on the trunk or pelvis that have not improved within 30 days on a Group 1 product
- a requirement for a continuation of therapy from hospital or nursing home for recent ulcer, flap, or graft procedures (surgery within the past 60 days)

GROUP 3

These products are air-fluidized beds. Patients must have *all* of the following characteristics:

- Stage III or IV pressure ulcer on trunk or pelvis
- bedridden/severe immobility
- required institutionalization without air-fluidized bed
- physician order and monthly rectification
- care plan/assessment
- Group 2 product tried without success
- trained adult caregiver available

- moderate depletion 5 5–10 mg/dl
- severe depletion, 5 mg/dl
- Nutritional Risk Screening Form (Exhibit 6–3)
- 3-day intake diary
- weight loss (may be difficult to assess in bedbound patient due to lack of bed scales in the home)

For at-risk patients (adapt to the individual needs of the patient)

- Increase intake (add supplements, high-protein milk, powdered milk, eggs, peanut butter, cheese).
- Increase caloric intake (small frequent feedings, butter, creams, fats, sugars).
- Encourage fluids.
- Add multivitamin with minerals.

TIP Serum albumin levels may not be representative of the current nutritional status due to a half-life of approximately 20 days. If available, prealbumin levels are a more accurate marker in nutritional status.

Consult a clinical dietitian as needed.

Skin Care

Maintain clean, soft, supple skin.

Bathing

- Schedule baths based on patient need.
- Use mild soaps.
- Use moisturizers.

Incontinence

- Always evaluate for etiology and treat appropriately.
- Cleanse immediately using products designed for perineal care.
- Protect skin from the next episode of incontinence with the use of moisture barriers.
- Minimize use of diapers; use only when patient is out of bed.
- One open underpad on the bed should be sufficient when the patient is in bed.

Education

- Education must be patient specific.
- Patient and caregiver must be active participants.
- Multidisciplinary approaches may be needed, including:
  - physical therapy
  - occupational therapy
  - speech therapy
  - nutritional services
  - social services
- Instructions should be verbal and written at the patient and caregiver's level of understanding (see Appendix 6–A).
- Patients and caregivers should provide demonstrations to show understanding of teaching provided and verbalize a willingness to follow through on the developed plan of care.
- Monitor, on all patients, any variance. For example, home care–and skilled nursing facility–acquired pressure ulcers should be logged, tracked, and reported in compliance with agency policy.

> **TIP** Case management of at-risk patients is essential. Communication between the patient, caregiver, and staff involved is imperative, as is consistency with adherence to the developed plan of care.

TREATMENT CHOICES

Goals

- Prevent further breakdown.
- Reduce risk factors.
- Utilize appropriate topical therapy.
- Utilize appropriate adjunct therapy.

Pressure Redistribution

Group 2 mattresses are for treatment only, not prevention. Group 2 mattresses are:
- mattress replacements
- alternating air or low-air-loss mattresses

Patients must meet certain criteria to qualify for reimbursement of the mattress cost.

Group 3 mattresses are air-fluidized therapy. Patients must meet criteria for reimbursement.

Patient Movement

Patients must not be positioned on a pressure ulcer. If there are no turning surfaces without breakdown, the patient must be turned hourly and must be on a Group 2 or 3 mattress.

Nutrition

Maintain adequate nutrition that is compatible with the individual's wishes or condition. Consult with a clinical dietitian. See Exhibit 6–3.

Skin Care

Incontinence

Measures should be taken to avoid contamination of a wound from episodes of incontinence. Precautions include:

- occlusive dressings if indicated
- Foley catheters
- fecal incontinence devices
- bowel and bladder programs

Periwound Skin

Use protective skin barrier wipes.

Local Wound Treatment

- Cleanse or irrigate with normal saline.
- Choose the optimum category of wound product based on stage, location, and assessment of the wound.
- Locate information about wound treatments.

TIP Once a pressure ulcer has closed, the site remains extremely vulnerable to repeat breakdown. Aggressive measures are needed to prevent recurrence.

CASE STUDY

Mr. Brown is a 68-year-old male admitted to home care following a cerebral vascular accident with resultant left-sided paralysis and swallowing difficulties. He has an indwelling Foley catheter for neurogenic bladder and has occasionally been incontinent of stool. His Braden Scale score is 14, showing a moderate risk for skin breakdown. His wife, age 65, is a homemaker and a willing and able caregiver. One daughter lives nearby; a son lives 2 hours away. The home is considered to be clean, tidy, and adequate for care.

A multidisciplinary approach was taken to plan Mr. Brown's care. The RN case manager led the team. It included a physical therapist to assist/instruct in transfers and strengthening, an occupational therapist to instruct in maximizing resumption of activities of daily living, a speech therapist to assess and assist with swallowing problems, a social worker for community resources and respite care, and a home health aide to assist with personal care.

Medical equipment ordered included a hospital bed with a Group 1 mattress replacement, a trapeze, a bedside commode, a wheelchair, and a therapeutic foam seating cushion.

The RN instructed Mr. and Mrs. Brown in the importance of maintaining skin integrity through positioning, nutrition, and routine skin care. Together they constructed a schedule that was acceptable to all involved.

After 2 months of care and instructions, Mrs. Brown felt able to care for her spouse with a monthly visit from the RN to change the Foley and reassess the patient's status. She continued to have a home health aide three times weekly to assist with bathing and personal care (this also gave Mrs. Brown time to shop and tend to her needs).

Mr. Brown did not develop any pressure ulcers in a 1-year period from the time of his admission to home care.

Mr. Brown's Schedule

8 AM	Up in wheelchair for breakfast
9 AM	Toileting regimen
10 AM	Bath:
	• Monday, Wednesday, Friday by home health aide
	• Tuesday and Thursday by spouse
	• Saturday and Sunday by daughter
11 AM	Bed, right side
Noon	Lunch, in bed with head of bed elevated
1 PM	Nap on left side
3:30 PM	Up in wheelchair to watch TV, weight shifts with each commercial break
5 PM	Dinner in wheelchair
6 PM	Toileting, then in recliner chair for reading or TV
9 PM	Bed, on back with head of bed not elevated over 30∞, range-of-motion exercises performed
10 PM	Snack (high protein) with head of bed elevated
10:30 PM	Right side with pillow supports for back and knees
2:30 AM	Pillows removed, on back
6:30 AM	Draw sheet used to turn to left side, one small pillow for support

The AHCPR Pressure Ulcer Treatment Guidelines for the Patient were utilized in instructing the caregiver. (See Appendix 6–A.)

BIBLIOGRAPHY

Ayello, E. A., & Draden, B. (2002, May/June). How and why to do pressure ulcer risk assessment. *Advances in Skin and Wound Care, 15*(3), 125–132.

Baharestani, M. (1999). Pressure ulcers in an age of managed care: A nursing perspective. *Ostomy/Wound Management, 45*(5), 18–40.

Beck, F. K., & Rosenthal, T. C. (2002, April). Prealbumin: A marker for nutritional evaluation. *American Family Physician, 16*(8), 1575–1578.

Blaszcyk, J. (1998). Make a difference: Standardize your heel care practice. *Ostomy/Wound Management, 44*(5), 32–40.

Cali, T. G. et al. (1999). Pressure ulcer treatment: Examining selected costs of therapeutic failure. *Advanced Wound Care, 12*(Suppl. 2), 8–11.

Haalboom, J. (1999). Risk-assessment tools in the prevention of pressure ulcers. *Ostomy/Wound Management, 45*(2), 20–34.

Maklebust, J., & Sieggreen, M. (1996). *Pressure ulcers: Guidelines for prevention and nursing management* (2d ed.). Springhouse, PA: Springhouse Corp.

National Pressure Ulcer Advisory Panel. (2007). Pressure ulcer stages revised by NPUAP. Retrieved October 8, 2011, from http://www.npuap.org/pr2.htm.

Peiper, B. (2007). Mechanical forces: Pressure, sheer and friction. In R. A. Bryant & D. P. Nix (Eds.), *Acute and chronic wounds, Current management concepts* (3rd ed., pp. 205–234). St. Louis, MO. Mosby Elsevier.

Provo, B. et al. (1997). Practice versus knowledge when it comes to pressure ulcer prevention. *Journal of Wound, Ostomy, and Continence Nursing, 24*, 265–269.

Stotts, N., & Cavanaugh, C. (1999). Assessing the patient with a wound. *Home Health Care Nurse, 17*(1), 27–35.

Van Rijswijk, L., & Braden, B. (1999). Pressure ulcer patient and wound assessment: An AHCPR clinical practice guideline update. *Ostomy/Wound Management, 45*(Suppl. 1A), 565–675.

Yastrub, D. J. (2010). Pressure or pathology: Distinguishing pressure ulcers from the Kennedy Terminal Ulcer. *Journal of Wound, Ostomy, and Continence Nursing, 37*(3), 249–250.

Patient Guide: AHCPR Pressure Ulcer Treatment Guidelines for the Patient

A pressure sore is serious. It must not be ignored. With proper treatment, most pressure sores will heal. Healing depends on many things: your general health, diet, relieving pressure on the sore, and careful cleaning and dressing of the sore. Share this handout with your family members and caregivers. By working with healthcare professionals and following these guidelines, you and your caregiver can better treat pressure sores and prevent new ones.

This handout will help you and your caregiver care for pressure sores. It also gives basic information about preventing new sores.

This handout gives the steps essential to helping a pressure sore heal. Although not all steps apply to everyone, it is important that you:

- Learn how to prevent and treat pressure sores.
- Ask questions if you do not understand.
- Explain your needs and concerns.
- Know what is best for you.
- Be active in your care.

TREATMENT

Healing a pressure sore is a team effort. A team of healthcare professionals will work with you to prepare a treatment plan. Your team may include doctors, nurses, dietitians, social workers, pharmacists, and occupational and physical therapists. However, you and your caregiver are the most important team members. Feel free to ask questions or share concerns with other team members.

Your Role

You and your caregiver need to:

- Know your roles in the treatment program.
- Learn how to perform the care.
- Know what to report to the physician or nurse.
- Know how to tell if the treatment works.
- Help change the treatment plan when needed.
- Know what questions you want to ask.
- Get answers you understand.

Treatment Plan

To develop a treatment plan that meets your needs, the physician or nurse must know about

- your general health.
- illnesses that might slow healing (such as diabetes or hardening of the arteries).
- prescription or over-the-counter medicines you take.
- the emotional support and physical assistance available from family, friends, and others.

Your physician or nurse will perform a physical exam and check the condition of your pressure sore to decide how to care for it. If you have had a pressure sore before, tell the physician or nurse what helped it heal and what didn't help.

Your emotional health is also important. Be sure to share information about stresses in your life as well as health beliefs and practices. This will help your care team design a treatment plan that meets your personal needs.

The treatment plan will be based on the results of your physical exam, health history, personal circumstances, and the condition of the sore (how it looks). This plan will include specific instructions for

- taking pressure off the sore.
- caring for the pressure sore by cleaning the wound, removing dead tissue and debris, and dressing or bandaging the area to protect it while it heals.
- aiding healing by making sure you get enough calories, protein, vitamins, and minerals.

Note to Caregivers

Although patients should be as active in their care as possible, you may need to provide much or all of their care. As a result, you may find you have questions or problems. If so, ask for help. Call physicians, nurses, and other professionals for answers and other support.

Remember that patients who must be in a bed or chair for long periods don't have to get pressure sores. Pressure sores can be prevented, and sores that have formed can be healed.

Helping Pressure Sores Heal

Healing pressure sores depends on three principles: pressure relief, care of the sore, and good nutrition.

PRESSURE RELIEF

Pressure sores form when there is constant pressure on certain parts of the body. Long periods of unrelieved pressure cause or worsen pressure sores and slow healing once a sore has formed. Taking pressure off the sore is the first step toward healing.

Pressure sores usually form on parts of the body over bony prominences (such as hips and heels) that bear weight when you sit or lie down for a long time. **Figure 6–A1** shows "pressure points" where sores often form.

You can relieve or reduce pressure by

- using special surfaces to support your body.
- putting your body in certain positions.
- changing positions often.

Support Surfaces

Support surfaces are special beds, mattresses, mattress overlays, or seat cushions that support your body in bed or in a chair. These surfaces reduce or relieve pressure. By relieving pressure, you can help pressure sores heal and prevent new ones from forming.

You can get different kinds of support surfaces. The best kind depends on your general health, if you are able to change positions, your body build, and the condition of your sore. You and your physician or nurse can choose the surface that is best for you.

One way to see if a support surface reduces pressure enough is for the caregiver to do a "hand check" under the person (**Figure 6–A2**). The caregiver places his or her hand under the support surface, beneath the pressure point, with the palm up and fingers flat. If there is less than one inch of support surface between the pressure point of the body and the caregiver's

Figure 6–A1. Pressure Points. Dots show pressure points when lying on back (A), when sitting (B), and when lying on side (C).

Figure 6–A2 Hand Check to Assess Pressure Relief. Slide hand (palm up and fingers flat) under support surface, just under pressure point. Do not flex fingers.

hand, the surface does not give enough support. If you need more support, your physician or nurse will recommend a different support surface.

Caregivers should know that pressure sores are often painful, and a hand check may increase pain. Caregivers should ask if it will be okay to do a hand check, which should be done as gently as possible.

Good Body Positions

Your position is important to relieving pressure on the sore and preventing new ones. You need to switch positions whether you are in a bed or a chair.

In Bed

Follow these guidelines:

- Do not lie on the pressure sore. Use foam pads or pillows to relieve pressure on the sore, as shown in **Figure 6–A3**.
- Change position at least every 2 hours.
- Do not rest directly on your hip bone when lying on your side. A 30-degree, sidelying position is best (Figure 6–A3).
- When lying on your back, keep your heels up off the bed by placing a thin foam pad or pillow under your legs from midcalf to ankle (**Figure 6–A4**). The pad or pillow should raise the heels just enough so a piece of paper can be passed between them and the bed. Do not place the pad or pillow directly under the knee when on your back because this could reduce blood flow to your lower leg.
- Do not use donut-shaped (ring) cushions—they reduce blood flow to tissue.
- Use pillows or small foam pads to keep knees and ankles from touching each other.
- Raise the head of the bed as little as possible. Raise it no more than 30 degrees from horizontal (**Figure 6–A5**). If you have other health problems (such as respiratory ail-

Figure 6–A3 Best Position While on Side.

Figure 6–A4 Keep Heels off Bed.

Figure 6–A5 Head of Bed Raised 30 Degrees.

ments) that are improved by sitting up, ask your doctor or nurse which positions are best.

- Use the upright position during meals to prevent choking. The head of the bed can be moved back to a lying or semireclining position 1 hour after eating.

In a Chair or Wheelchair

When sitting, you should have good posture and be able to keep upright in the chair or wheelchair (**Figure 6–A6**). A good position will allow you to move more easily and help prevent new sores.

For your specific needs, use cushions designed to relieve pressure on sitting surfaces. Even if pressure can be relieved with cushions, your position should be changed every hour. Remember to:

- Avoid sitting directly on the pressure sore.
- Keep the top of your thighs horizontal and your ankles in a comfortable, "neutral" position on the floor or footrest (Figure 6–A6). Rest your elbows, forearms, and wrists on arm supports.

Figure 6–A6 Best Position While Sitting.

- If you cannot move yourself, have someone help you change your position at least every hour. If you can move yourself, shifting your weight every 15 minutes is even better.
- If your position in a chair cannot be changed, have someone help you back to bed so you can change position.
- Do not use donut-shaped or ring cushions because they reduce blood flow to tissue.

Changing Positions

Change your body position often—at least every hour while seated in a chair and at least every 2 hours while lying in bed. A written turning schedule or a turn clock (with positions written next to times) may help you and your caregiver remember turning times and positions. You may want to set a kitchen timer.

Be sure your plan works for you. It should consider your skin's condition, personal needs and preferences, and your comfort level.

PRESSURE SORE CARE

The second principle of healing is proper care of the sore. The three aspects of care are:

- cleaning
- removing dead tissue and debris (debridement)
- dressing (bandaging) the pressure sore

Pressure sore care is summarized in **Table 6–A1**. You should know about sore care even if only your caregiver is caring for the sore. Knowing about your care will help you make informed decisions about it.

Cleaning

Pressure sores heal best when they are clean. They should be free of dead tissue (which may look like a scab), excess fluid draining from the sore, and other debris. If not, healing can be slowed, and infection can result.

A healthcare professional will show you and your caregiver how to clean and/or rinse the pressure sore. Clean the sore each time dressings are changed.

Cleaning usually involves rinsing, or "irrigating," the sore. Loose material may also be gently wiped away with a gauze pad. It is important to use the right equipment and methods for cleaning the sore. Tissue that is healing can be hurt if too much force is used when rinsing. Cleaning may be ineffective if too little force is used.

Use only cleaning solutions recommended by a healthcare professional. Usually saline is best for rinsing the pressure sore. Saline can be bought at a drug store or made at home (see **Table 6–A2**).

Caution: Sometimes water supplies become contaminated. If the health department warns against drinking the water, use saline from the drug store or use bottled water to make saline for cleaning sores.

Table 6–A1 Basic Steps of Pressure Sore Care

Task	Steps
Prepare	1. Wash hands with soap and water. 2. Get supplies: saline; irrigation equipment (syringe or other device, basin, large plastic bag); dressings and tape; disposable plastic gloves and small plastic (sandwich) bag; towel; glasses, goggles, and plastic apron (optional). 3. Move patient into comfortable position. 4. Place large plastic bag on bed to protect bed linen.
Remove dressing	1. Place hand into small plastic bag (Figure 6–A7). 2. Grasp old dressing with bag-covered hand and pull off dressing. 3. Turn bag inside out over the old dressing. 4. Close the bag tightly before throwing it away.
Irrigate the sore	1. Put on disposable plastic gloves. (Wear glasses or goggles and plastic apron if drainage might splash.) 2. Fill syringe or other device with saline. 3. Place basin under pressure sore to catch drainage. 4. Hold irrigation device 1 to 6 inches from sore and spray it with saline. Use enough force to remove dead tissue and old drainage but not enough to damage new tissue. 5. Carefully remove basin so fluid doesn't spill. 6. Dry the skin surrounding the sore by patting skin with soft, clean towel. 7. After assessing and dressing the sore, remove gloves by pulling them inside out. Throw away gloves properly.
Assess the sore	1. Assess healing. As sore heals, it will slowly become smaller and drain less. New tissue at the bottom of the sore is light red or pink and looks lumpy and glossy. Do not disturb this tissue. 2. Tell health care provider if the sore is larger, drainage increases, the sore is infected, or there are no signs of healing in 2 to 4 weeks.
Dress the sore	Place a new dressing over the sore as instructed by the physician or nurse. Remember to: • Use dressings only once. • Keep dressings in the original package or other closed plastic package. • Store dressings in a clean, dry place. • Throw out the entire package if any dressings get wet, contaminated, or dirty. • Wash your hands before touching clean dressings. • Do not touch packaged dressings once you touch the sore.

Table 6–A2 Recipe for Making Saline (Salt Water)

1. Use 1 gallon of distilled water or boil 1 gallon of tap water for 5 minutes. Do not use well water or seawater. Be sure storage container and mixing utensil are clean (boiled).
2. Add 8 teaspoons of table salt to the distilled or boiled water.
3. Mix the solution well until the salt is completely dissolved.

Note: Cool to room temperature before using. This solution can be stored at room temperature in a tightly covered glass or plastic bottle for up to 1 week.

Do not use antiseptics such as hydrogen peroxide or iodine. They can damage sensitive tissue and prevent healing.

Cleansing methods are usually effective in keeping sores clean. However, in some cases, other methods will be needed to remove dead tissue.

Removing Dead Tissue and Debris

Dead tissue in the pressure sore can delay healing and lead to infection. Removing dead tissue is often painful. You may want to take pain-relieving medicine 30 to 60 minutes before these procedures.

Under supervision of healthcare professionals, dead tissue and debris can be removed in several ways:

- rinsing (to wash away loose debris)
- wet-to-dry dressings. In this special method, wet dressings are put on and allowed to dry. Dead tissue and debris are pulled off when the dry dressing is taken off. This method is only used to remove dead tissue; it is never used on a clean wound.
- enzyme medications to dissolve dead tissue only
- special dressings left in place for several days help the body's natural enzymes dissolve dead tissue slowly. This method should not be used if the sore is infected. With infected sores, a faster method for removing dead tissue and debris should be used.

Qualified healthcare professionals may use surgical instruments to cut away dead tissue.

Based on the person's general health and the condition of the sore, the physician or nurse will recommend the best method for removing dead tissue.

Choosing and Using Dressings

Choosing the right dressings is important to pressure sore care. The physician or nurse will consider the location and condition of the pressure sore when recommending dressings.

The most common dressings are gauze (moistened with saline), film (see-through), and hydrocolloid (moisture- and oxygen-retaining) dressings. Gauze dressings must be moistened often with saline and changed at least daily. If they are not kept moist, new tissue will be pulled off when the dressing is removed.

Unless the sore is infected, film or hydrocolloid dressings can be left on for several days to retain the sore's natural moisture.

The choice of dressing is based on

- the type of material that will best aid healing.
- how often dressings will need to be changed.
- whether the sore is infected.

In general, the dressing should keep the sore moist and the surrounding skin dry. As the sore heals, a different type of dressing may be needed.

Storing and Caring for Dressings

Clean (rather than sterile) dressings usually can be used if they are kept clean and dry. There is no evidence that using sterile dressings is better than using clean dressings. However, contamination between patients can occur in hospitals and nursing homes. When clean dressings are used in institutions, procedures that prevent cross-contamination should be followed carefully.

At home, clean dressings may also be used. Carefully follow the methods given here on how to store, care for, and change dressings.

To keep dressings clean and dry:

- Store dressings in their original packages (or in other protective, closed plastic packages) in a clean, dry place.
- Wash hands with soap and water before touching clean dressings.
- Take dressings from the box only when they will be used.
- Do not touch the packaged dressing once the sore has been touched.
- Discard the entire package if any dressings become wet or dirty.

Changing Dressings

Ask your physician or nurse to show you how to remove dressings and put on new ones. If possible, he or she should watch you change the dressings at least once.

Ask for written instructions if you need them. Discuss any problems or questions about changing dressings with the physician or nurse.

Wash your hands with soap and water before and after each dressing change. Use each dressing only once. You should check to be sure the dressing stays in place when changing positions. After the used dressing is removed, it must be disposed of safely to prevent the spread of germs that may be on dressings.

Using Plastic Bags for Removal

A small plastic bag (such as a sandwich bag) can be used to lift the dressing off the pressure sore (**Figure 6–A7**). Seal the bag before throwing it away. If you use gloves, throw them away after each use.

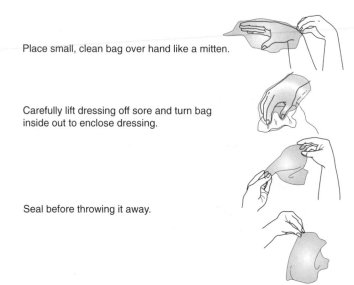

Place small, clean bag over hand like a mitten.

Carefully lift dressing off sore and turn bag
inside out to enclose dressing.

Seal before throwing it away.

Figure 6–A7 Plastic Bag Method of Removing Bandages.

GOOD NUTRITION

Good nutrition is the third principle of healing. Eating a balanced diet will help your pressure
sore heal and prevent new sores from forming.

You and your physician, dietitian, or nurse should review any other medical conditions you
have (such as diabetes or kidney problems) before designing a special diet.

Weigh yourself weekly. If you find you cannot eat enough food to maintain your weight or
if you notice a sudden increase or decrease, you may need a special diet and vitamin supplements. You may need extra calories as part of a well-balanced diet.

Tell your physician or nurse about any weight change. An unplanned weight gain or loss of
10 pounds or more in 6 months should be looked into.

PAIN AND INFECTION

Even if you care for your pressure sore properly, problems may come up. Pain and infection are
two such problems. Pain can make it hard to move or to participate in care. Infection can slow
healing.

Managing Pain

You may feel pain in or near the pressure sore. Tell your physician or nurse if you do. Covering
the sore with a dressing or changing your body position may lessen the pain.

If you feel pain during cleaning of the pressure sore or during dressing changes, medicine
may help. It may be over-the-counter or prescription medicine. Take medicine to relieve pain

30 to 60 minutes before these procedures to give it time to work. Tell your physician or nurse if your pain medicine does not work.

Treating Infection

Healing may slow if the sore becomes infected. Infection from the sore can spread to surrounding tissue (cellulitis), to underlying bone (osteomyelitis), or throughout the body (sepsis). These serious complications demand immediate medical attention. If you notice any of the signs of infection as described in **Table 6–A3**, call your physician right away.

CHECKING YOUR PROGRESS

A healthcare professional should check your pressure sore regularly. How often depends on how well the sore is healing. Generally, a pressure sore should be checked weekly.

Examining the Sore

The easiest time to check pressure sores is after cleaning. Signs of healing include decreased size and depth of the sore and less drainage. You should see signs of healing in 2 to 4 weeks. Infected sores may take longer to heal.

Signs to Report

Tell your physician or nurse if:

- The pressure sore is larger or deeper.
- More fluid drains from the sore.
- The sore does not begin to heal in 2 to 4 weeks.
- You see signs of infection (Table 6–A3).

Also report if:

- You cannot eat a well-balanced diet.
- You have trouble following any part of the treatment plan.
- Your general health becomes worse.

Table 6–A3 Signs of Infection

Infected Sore	Widespread Infection
Thick green or yellow drainage	Fever or chills
Foul odor	Weakness
Redness or warmth around sore	Confusion or difficulty concentrating
Tenderness of surrounding area	Rapid heartbeat
Swelling	

Changing the Treatment Plan

If any of these signs exist, you and your healthcare professional may need to change the treatment plan. Depending on your needs, these factors may be changed:

- support surfaces
- how often you change how you sit or lie
- methods of cleaning and removing dead tissue
- type of dressing
- nutrition
- infection treatment

Other Treatment Choices

If sores do not heal, your physician may recommend electrotherapy. A very small electrical current is used to stimulate healing in this procedure. This is a fairly new treatment for pressure sores. Proper equipment and trained personnel may not always be available.

If your pressure sore is large or deep, or if it does not heal, surgery may be needed to repair damaged tissue. You and your physician can discuss possible surgery.

CARE OF HEALTHY SKIN

Having healthy skin is important to preventing future pressure sores. Healthy skin is less likely to be damaged and heals faster than skin in poor condition.

You can help prevent new pressure sores while helping to heal the ones you have. To improve your skin's health:

- Bathe when needed for cleanliness and comfort.
- Use mild soap and warm (not hot) water.
- Apply moisturizers (such as skin lotions) to keep skin from becoming too dry.

Inspect your skin at least once a day for redness or color changes or for sores. Pay special attention to pressure points where pressure sores can form (Figure 6–A1).

Skin problems can also result from bladder or bowel leakage (urinary or fecal incontinence). If you have these problems, ask your physician or nurse for help. If the leakage cannot be controlled completely, you should:

- Clean your skin as soon as it becomes soiled.
- Use a protective cream or ointment on the skin to protect it from wetness.
- Use incontinence pads and/or briefs to absorb wetness away from the skin.

For more detailed information about how to prevent pressure sores, ask for a copy of *Preventing Pressure Ulcers: Patient Guide.*

FOR MORE INFORMATION

Information in this handout is based on *Treatment of Pressure Ulcers, Clinical Practice Guideline*, No. 15. It was developed by a nonfederal panel sponsored by the Agency for Healthcare Research and Quality (AHRQ), formerly known as the Agency for Health Care Policy and Research (AHCPR), an agency of the Public Health Service.

BE ACTIVE IN YOUR CARE

If you understand the basic ideas of pressure relief, sore care, and good nutrition, you can take the steps needed to heal pressure sores and prevent new ones. Not all steps apply to every person. The best program will be based on your needs and the condition of your sores.

Be sure to:

- Ask questions.
- Explain your needs, wants, and concerns.
- Understand what is being done and why.
- Know what is best for you. Discuss what you can do to prevent and treat pressure sores—at home, in the hospital, or in the nursing home.

Being active in your care can mean better care.

ADDITIONAL RESOURCES

The following organizations offer a variety of resources for people who are concerned about pressure sores.

Booklets and Information for Patients, Caregivers, and Families Providing Care at Home

U.S. Department of Health and Human Services Public Health Service Agency for Health Care Research and Quality. www.ahrq.gov

Link to Appendix 6–A (printed in this chapter) AHCPR, *Pressure Ulcer Treatment Guideline*: http://www.ncbi.nlm.nih.gov/books/NBK63915/ This guideline is currently out of print, and listed by the AHCPR as out of date. However, there is no replacement document at this time that is user friendly for patients or caregivers. The principles described here are straightforward and easy to follow steps to prevent and/or treat pressure ulcers.

Information about Nutrition

National Center for Nutrition and Dietetics (NCND)
National Pressure Ulcer Advisory Panel (NPUAP) serves as the authoritative voice for improved patient outcomes in pressure ulcer prevention and treatment through public policy, education and research. www.npuap.org

Arterial Ulcers

Julie Phelps Maloy

Arterial ulcers, usually located on the distal lower extremity, can be either acute or chronic. They have a round, punched out shape and a pale wound bed. They indicate a severe reduction or elimination of oxygenated blood flow to the leg or foot that has resulted in tissue ischemia and/or necrosis (**Figure 7–1**; **Color Plate 14**). The lack of oxygen to the tissue causes leg and/or foot pain for the patient. It is important to determine the type of pain the patient is experiencing. Is it burning, aching, or cramping? Is the pain constant or intermittent? Pain that is exercise induced is referred to as intermittent claudication. Rest pain can be an indication of a threatened limb (Siegel, 1998, p. 125). Some studies find that approximately 21% of all lower extremity ulcers have some form of arterial involvement. Precipitating factors include diabetes, smoking, hypertension, and hypercholesterolemia (Rubano & Kerstein, 1998, p. 147). The precipitating event leading to the ulceration is not always known but can result from progressive vessel occlusion or from trauma that leads to an increase in oxygen demands. Arterial disease and tissue ischemia set the stage, trauma occurs, and an ulcer results. Topical treatments are always important in chronic wound care; however, in ischemic ulcers, increased blood flow to the area through surgical intervention is the only effective way to heal the ulcer. Complications include infection, gangrene, and death. It is extremely important for the nurse to know if there is arterial involvement in a lower extremity ulcer (**Figure 7–2**; **Color Plate 15**). Without understanding the underlying cause of the ulcer, frustration results for the nurse and probable complications result for the patient.

ETIOLOGY

Arterial ulcers result from lack of blood supply, which can stem from several factors:

- Atherosclerosis is the most common cause. Plaque forms on the walls of the arteries, causing a narrowing of the lumen and decreased

Figure 7–1 Arterial Ulcers. Note dry, flaky skin and absence of hair.

Clinical Objectives:

(1) Protect

(2) Clean

(3) Provide moisture cautiously

(4) Provide comfort

See Color Plate 14.

Figure 7–2 Ischemic Foot with Gangrene. Do not initiate topical treatment. Notify physician of status and any changes immediately.

See Color Plate 15.

blood flow. Plaque formation can lead to thrombosis, embolization, and ischemia.

- Arterial embolism, when the body has no time to develop collateral circulation to compensate with resulting ischemia
- Vasospastic disease (e.g., Raynaud disease)
- Trauma (open and/or closed injuries)
- Diabetes mellitus

ASSESSMENT

Risk Factors

- hypertension
- smoking
- diabetes mellitus
- hyperlipidemia
- male gender (males are more at risk than females)
- history of angina, myocardial infarction, or cerebrovascular accident

Clinical Signs

See Holloway (1997, pp. 158–172) for comparison charts with venous insufficiency, arterial insufficiency, and peripheral neuropathy.

Wound

- uniform wound edges, a punched out appearance
- small in size but can be superficial or deep
- pale wound bed (due to the lack of oxygenated blood in the area) can also be gray or yellow with no new tissue
- limited or no surrounding inflammation
- minimal drainage
- necrosis (frequently present)
- loss of hair at the ankle or foot
- surrounding skin can appear shiny and tight

Location

Arterial ulcers are commonly found on the distal extremity. They can be above the malleoli; however, they are frequently found below, on the toe joints and/or lateral border of the foot. Trauma from footwear is a frequent cause of the ulcer formation.

> **TIP** When a wound is obscured by necrotic tissue or is purple and indurated, document it as "unable to stage, consistent with deeper tissue damage."

Pain

- burning, cramping, or weariness located in the calf, thigh, buttocks, or foot
- located in foot when resting, particularly at night, indicating severe occlusion and a threatened limb
- increases with leg elevation
- increases with walking due to a lack of oxygen delivery to the working leg muscles (intermittent claudication) and can diminish within 1 to 5 minutes after the exertion is stopped
- usually focused distal to the point of occlusion in the vessel
- can be masked in the diabetic patient due to neuropathy
- can sometimes be relieved by a dependent leg position

Other Clinical Signs

- pallor of extremity on elevation
- dependent rubor of the extremity
- thickened, yellow, fragile nails
- pulses palpable or not palpable in the dorsalis pedis and posterior tibialis
- dorsalis pedis: Use the second and third fingers to palpate the pulse on the dorsum of the foot. Place your thumb on the plantar surface of the foot to steady your hand. Use a light touch to avoid occluding the artery.
- posterior tibialis: Palpate lightly posterior to the medial malleolus using the second and third fingers. Place your thumb on the lateral malleolus.
- foot cool or cold to touch
- absence of hair on the leg
- history of trauma to the foot or leg

Complications

- wound infection (Local signs can include erythema, edema, warmth, induration, increased pain, and purulent and/or an increase in wound exudate.)
- gangrene
- amputation
- death

TREATMENT CHOICES

Goal

The goal is to establish adequate circulation to the affected area. (Ulcers associated with ischemia heal when the blood supply is reestablished.)

Diagnostics

Several systems can be used to confirm and locate perfusion problems.

- Noninvasive studies of the arterial system can be performed using an ultra-sonic Doppler to determine the ankle-brachial index (ABI) (Falanga, 1997, pp. 169–170) (**Exhibit 7–1**).
- A normal ABI is considered to be 0.9–1.1.
- Claudication can occur between 0.5 and 0.6.
- Tissue loss and rest pain (signaling a threatened limb) can occur at < 0.5.

Most people consider an ABI to be invalid in a diabetic patient. The increased atherosclerosis with resulting calcified vessels may cause a falsely elevated ABI.

- Segmental pressures help locate the site or sites of occlusion by a decrease in the pressure.
- Vascular laboratories can do transcutaneous oxygen measurements (tcpO$_2$) to help determine the degree of microvascular perfusion.
- A reading of < 20 mm Hg indicates marked ischemia that will not heal.
- A reading of > 30 mm Hg indicates that healing can occur. Readings are not valid in the presence of a wound infection.

Surgical Intervention for Revascularization

Indications include rest pain, ischemic ulceration, and gangrene. This disease is progressive; without surgery or with unsuccessful surgery, gangrene and amputation can occur within a relatively short period of time (from a few weeks to a few months).

Medical Management

Nonsurgical candidates require good wound care and patient education. Pentoxifylline (Trental®) is used with some patients who are not experiencing resting pain. (There is controversy on its value for these patients.) Nurses should recognize that this is a progressive condition that can advance either slowly or rapidly.

Local Wound Management

- Clean the wound with normal saline or a commercially prepared wound cleanser.
- Removing eschar from heels and toes that have no symptoms of infection, leakage of exudate, or odor increases the opportunity for infection and can

Exhibit 7–1 Ankle-Brachial Index

Definition: An ankle-brachial index (ABI) is a noninvasive Doppler test for determining the presence and severity of arterial occlusive disease by calculating the ratio of the systolic pressure at the ankle to the systolic pressure in the brachial artery in the arm (Siegel, 1998, p. 129; Steed, 1997, p. 173).

EQUIPMENT

1. Doppler probe (ultrasound stethoscope)
2. blood pressure cuff
   - Make sure the cuff size is appropriate for the arm size. A cuff that is too short or too narrow can give falsely high readings. The inflatable bladder of the cuff should have a width of about 40% of the upper arm circumference. The length of the bladder should be about 80% of the arm circumference.
   - A regular cuff on an obese arm can give a falsely high reading (Bickley & Hockelman, 1999, p. 291).
3. ultrasound gel

PROCEDURE (Morison et al., 1997, pp. 198–199)

1. The patient should lie flat for 15–20 minutes before obtaining pressure readings.
2. Apply the blood pressure cuff around the patient's arm, and apply ultrasound gel over the brachial pulse.
3. Hold the Doppler probe at a 45 degree angle, and place it over the brachial pulse.
4. When a good signal is obtained, inflate the cuff until the signal disappears and gradually deflate until the sound returns. The first sound heard is the systolic brachial pressure. Repeat in the other arm. Use the higher reading to calculate ABI.
5. Apply the cuff just above the ankle. Palpate the posterior tibial or dorsalis pedis pulse. Apply ultrasound gel.
6. Repeat steps 3 and 4.
7. $ABI = \dfrac{\text{ankle systolic pressure}}{\text{brachial systolic pressure}}$

INTERPRETATION

The ABI can be falsely elevated in those who have diabetes because there can be calcification of the inner layer of the arteries preventing the cuff from successfully compressing the arteries.

There are slight variations depending on the resource. Generally,

- 0.8–1.0 indicates that compression is an option for treatment: there is little or no arterial disease. (Some authorities will compress with 0.7.)
- If ABI equals 0.5–0.8, refer to a vascular specialist. The patient may be experiencing intermittent claudication. Compression is not indicated as a treatment option.
- At ≤ 0.5, refer to a vascular specialist. This is a threatened limb. Compression is contraindicated.

Systolic Doppler Pressures

	Brachial	Dorsalis Pedis	Posterior Tibial
Right	90	50	40
Left	100	0	100

Note: Always use the highest brachial pressure and the highest ankle pressure to calculate the ABI.

ABI = 50/100 = 0.5 in the right lower extremity; the highest ankle pressure is 50. Using the highest brachial pressure (which is the left arm), divide the 50 by 100, which equals 0.5.

ABI = 100/100 = 1.0 in the left lower extremity; the highest ankle pressure is 100. Using the left arm pressure again, divide the 100 at the ankle by the 100 brachial pressure, which equals 1.0.

TIPS
- Consider the whole patient and the etiology. It is easy to get caught up in wanting the wound to heal with topical treatments and to forget the true cause of the ulcer.
- Explain the etiology to the patient along with signs and symptoms of complications.
- Without revascularization, the wound will usually become a chronic nonhealing wound.

---

quickly lead to an amputation due to already compromised blood supply to the area (Doughty & Holbrook, 2007, pp. 277–278).
- Select a dressing that supports realistic healing goals for the wound.

PREVENTION

Patient Education

(See Appendix 7–A).

- Provide information on the underlying cause of the ulceration(s).
- Reinforce dietary/blood sugar control for the diabetic patient.
- Stress the importance of cessation of smoking.
- Stress weight control and a mild exercise program (both for weight control and to build collateral circulation). Recommend a low-fat diet.
- Educate about blood pressure management (include a referral to stress reduction/management classes), if appropriate.
- Provide pharmacologic education on drug interactions and reactions for patients who are on medication.
- Explain that support stockings and compression are contraindicated because they further constrict the arteries.

- In regard to foot care, instruct the patient to:
  - Wash, dry, and lubricate feet daily.
  - Check for cracks and reddened areas—report any cracks or sores to the physician.
  - Check the inside of each shoe before inserting the foot.
  - Avoid walking barefoot.
  - Have nail care done by a professional such as a podiatrist.
  - Wear correctly fitting shoes, preferably fit by an orthotist or pedorthist.
- Educate the patient to signs and symptoms of complications along with what to do should they occur (including when to contact the physician and/or go to the emergency department). Complications include:
  - increase in pain from intermittent claudication to resting pain
  - infection
  - increasing wound necrosis
  - gangrene

CASE STUDY

Sam Shell was referred to your agency from his physician's office. He is homebound with a painful, nonhealing ulcer of the left foot located slightly above the outer malleolus (ankle). His medical history includes recently diagnosed diabetes mellitus, managed by diet, and coronary heart disease. He is 65 years old, 5 feet 10 inches tall, and weighs 243 pounds. He quit smoking 4 years ago when he had coronary bypass surgery. He is a retired truck driver.

Sam tells you he bumped his leg on his lawn mower several months ago, and he hasn't been able to get the ulcer to heal. Recently, it has become larger. His treatment includes cleansing with hydrogen peroxide followed by the application of an antibiotic cream. He keeps it covered with a bandage. Sam tells you he used to spend more time in his yard, but now he only walks around his house because his legs and buttocks hurt when he walks very far. Sometimes he wakes up in the night with leg pain, and when he does, he finishes the night in his recliner chair. Keeping his leg in the dependent position at night seems to help the pain go away.

On physical assessment, you find a round ulcer measuring approximately 3.0 centimeters in circumference located slightly above the left lateral malleolus. The ulcer, although shallow, is a full-thickness wound. The wound bed is pale pink, edges are even with yellow fibrin clinging to the edges, no necrosis, and minimal serous exudate on the dressing that had been applied the day before. There is no odor or surrounding erythema. The dorsalis pedis and posterior tibialis are not palpable. The leg and foot, which have been in a dependent position for several hours, have a purple red color. The color changes to a pale pink when Sam raises his leg above his heart for a few minutes. When direct pressure is applied to the nail beds, the capillary refill takes longer than 3 seconds.

An ABI, done in the home, is 0.5. The complete wound assessment, including the ABI, is communicated to the primary care physician along with the recommendation for a vascular consult. The topical treatment that is selected is one that provides moist wound healing and is not indicated for heavily exudating wounds. A hydrogel or hydrocolloid are two possible options. Wound cleansing can include either normal saline or a wound cleanser. Should normal saline be the choice for cleansing, the psi of the delivery system must be considered. A hydrogel impregnated gauze is selected, and it is held in place with a Kerlix dressing. Sam's wife is instructed in wound care while Sam awaits his physician appointment. They are both instructed about the signs and symptoms of complications and when to call the physician.

Sam is a candidate for revascularization, which he promptly has. Following surgery, ulcer care is selected to provide moist wound healing. The ulcer will heal quickly due to the increase in blood to the leg and foot. Dietary instruction includes a diabetic diet with a focus on low fat. A light exercise program of walking is also included in his rehabilitation to assist with weight control and build any needed collateral circulation in his left leg. Sam is instructed not to use any compression or support stockings in the future due to his atherosclerosis.

Note: Although this was carried out in the home as part of the assessment for a baseline, the reliability of an ABI can be questioned and can give a falsely high reading since Sam is a recently diagnosed noninsulin-dependent diabetic. Due to the vessel disease that can be present in a diabetic, most consider an ABI to be inconclusive, requiring more sophisticated studies to determine blood flow.

REFERENCES

Bickley, L. S., & Hockelman, R. A. (1999). *Bates' guide to physical examination and history taking* (7th ed.). Philadelphia: Lippincott.

Doughty, D. B., & Holbrook, R. (2007). Lower-extremity ulcers of vascular etiology. In R. A. Bryant & D. P. Nix (Eds.). *Acute and chronic wounds: Current management concepts* (3rd ed., pp. 258–277). St. Louis, MO. Mosby Elsevier.

Falanga, V. (1997). Venous ulceration: Assessment, classification, and management. In D. Krasner & D. Kane (Eds.), *Chronic wound care: A clinical source book for healthcare professionals* (2d ed., pp. 169–170). Wayne, PA: Health Management Publications.

Holloway, G. A. (1997). Arterial ulcers: Assessment, classification, and management. In D. Krasner & D. Kane (Eds.), *Chronic wound care: A clinical source book for healthcare professionals* (2d ed., pp. 158–172). Wayne, PA: Health Management Publications.

Morison, M., et al. (1997). *Nursing management of chronic wounds* (2d ed., pp. 198–199). Philadelphia: Mosby.

Rubano, J. J., & Kerstein, M. D. (1998). Arterial insufficiency and vasculitides. *Journal of Wound, Ostomy, and Continence Nursing, 25*(3), 147–157.

Siegel, A. (1998). Noninvasive vascular testing. In C. Sussman & B. M. Bates-Jensen (Eds.), *Wound care: A collaborative practice manual for physical therapists and nurses* (pp. 127–135). Gaithersburg, MD: Aspen.

Steed, D. (1997). Diabetic wounds: Assessment, classification and management. In D. Krasner & D. Kane (Eds.), *Chronic wound care: A clinical source book for healthcare professionals* (2d ed., pp. 173–174). Wayne, PA: Health Management Publications.

BIBLIOGRAPHY

Doughty, D. B. (2011). WOC nurse consult: Painful lower extremity ulcers. *Journal of Wound, Ostomy, and Continence Nursing*, 38(3), 265–267.

Salcrido, R. C. (Ed.). (2001). Arterial vs. venous ulcers: Diagnosis and treatments. *Skin and Wound Care*, 14(3), 146.

Sieggreen, M. Y., & Kline, R. A. (2000). Vascular ulcers. In S. Baranoski & E. A. Ayello (Eds.), *Wound care essentials: Practice principles* (pp. 271–310) Philadelphia, PA: Lippincott Williams & Wilkins.

Sieggreen, M. Y., & Kline, R. A. (2004). Arterial insufficiency and ulceration: Diagnosis and treatment options. BNET, The CBS Interactive Business Network. Retrieved from: http://findarticles.com/p/articles/mi_qa3977/is_200406/ai_n9425021/

Wound, Ostomy and Continence Nurses Society. (2002). *Guidelines for management of wounds in patients with lower-extremity arterial disease*. Glenview, IL: Author.

Patient Guide: Guidelines for Patients with Peripheral Arterial Disease

WHAT IS PERIPHERAL ARTERIAL DISEASE?

Your circulatory system is made up of the heart, arteries, veins, and capillaries. The flow of blood through your body, which is needed to provide nourishment and oxygen to your cells, is your "circulation."

Your arteries carry oxygen-rich blood to all parts of your body. Normally, the blood flows easily through the arteries. In arterial disease, the arteries become narrowed or blocked, and the vessels cannot carry enough blood to the legs and feet.

If the blockage develops slowly, smaller arteries will develop over time and allow some blood to flow around the narrowed area. This is called "collateral circulation."

WHAT ARE THE SIGNS AND SYMPTOMS OF ARTERIAL DISEASE?

Signs and symptoms of decreased blood flow will involve changes in the way your legs and feet look and feel. You may experience:

- pain when walking
- pain at rest
- decrease in leg hair growth
- pallor (or paleness) of leg or foot when raised
- blue/red coloring of the foot
- numbness or tingling
- cool temperature of the skin
- sore or wound that will not heal

WHO IS AT RISK FOR DEVELOPING ARTERIAL DISEASE?

The more risk factors a person has, the more likely he or she will develop arterial disease. The risk factors for arterial disease include:

- smoking
- high blood pressure

- heart disease
- family history of arterial disease
- stress
- high cholesterol
- diabetes
- overweight
- age

HOW CAN ARTERIAL DISEASE BE CONTROLLED OR PREVENTED?

Arterial disease (atherosclerosis) cannot totally be cured or prevented, but you can control certain risk factors by changing your health habits.

Smoking

Tobacco in any form should be avoided. Nicotine causes the blood vessels to constrict, which prevents the normal amount of blood from reaching the organs and extremities and increases the risk of atherosclerosis. Smoking also decreases the amount of oxygen in the blood and may be associated with blood clot formation.

Diet

By reducing cholesterol and saturated fats in the diet, you may reduce the risk of atherosclerosis.

High Blood Pressure

Untreated high blood pressure (hypertension) adds to the workload of the heart and creates stress on the arteries. Have your blood pressure checked regularly and take medications as ordered by your physician. Your physician may suggest stress management classes or a self-restricted diet.

Diabetes

People with diabetes are especially prone to atherosclerosis. It is important to follow the recommendations of a healthcare team regarding diet, treatment, and medications.

Exercise

Mild, regular, or daily exercise aids in the control of atherosclerosis.

FOOT CARE

When blood flow to the legs is decreased, small injuries to the feet or toes may result in serious infections, sores, or tissue death (gangrene). You need to:

Hand mirror

- AVOID situations that might cause a foot injury.
- NEVER expose your feet to extreme heat or cold or to strong chemicals.
- WASH and dry your feet thoroughly, but do not soak.
- AVOID going barefoot.
- WEAR new shoes only for short periods of time.
- INSPECT your shoes. Check inside your shoes for any objects that could injure your feet.
- INSPECT your feet daily. This is especially important if you have diabetes and/or decreased sensation in your feet.
- USE a mirror if you have trouble seeing your feet. Ask someone to help you.
- CHECK for areas of redness, warmth, swelling, sores, or drainage.
- KEEP your feet clean and dry. Use a moisturizer daily.
- CUT toenails straight across and no shorter than the length of the toe. Round corners with a fine emery board.
- CORNS, calluses, and bunions should be treated by a physician or nurse.
- SPECIAL SHOES or inserts may reduce callus formation and promote control.

CONCLUSION

With recent advances in vascular surgery, atherosclerosis may be treated with a low risk of complications. Surgery may improve or remove symptoms and restore you to a more independent lifestyle. Surgery does not cure atherosclerosis. The disease process is still present. You can help to control this. A firm commitment to keep follow-up appointments with your physician and reduce risk factors will help to control further disease.

Venous Stasis Ulcers

Julie Phelps Maloy

Venous stasis ulcers are the most common type of lower leg ulcer and are a symptom of underlying venous disease (**Figures 8–1, 8–2, 8–3; Color Plates 16, 17, 18**). Many are long standing with duration of over a year, causing embarrassment and anxiety for the patient. Recurrence is common. Some studies have indicated that many of those with a venous ulcer have had their first ulceration before the age of 65 (Falanga, 1997, p. 165). A common complaint of the person with venous insufficiency is swelling, discomfort, and heaviness of their legs. Trauma is frequently reported as the initial cause of the ulceration. Typically, these ulcers are not painful; however, when mild discomfort is present, it is usually relieved by leg elevation. Severe, unrelieved pain is suggestive of a different etiology. It is not uncommon for the patient with a venous stasis ulcer to have a history of deep vein thrombosis or previous surgery for varicose veins. Treatment and preventive measures focus on improving venous blood flow and removing the impediments to wound healing. These goals cannot be successfully achieved without the understanding and cooperation of the patient.

ETIOLOGY

Normal Anatomy of the Venous System

Deep Veins

- carry blood under pressure back to the heart
- contain valves to prevent backflow of blood
- are located within the fascia

Superficial Veins

- carry blood under low pressure
- contain valves to prevent backflow of blood
- drain into deeper veins
- are located outside of the fascia

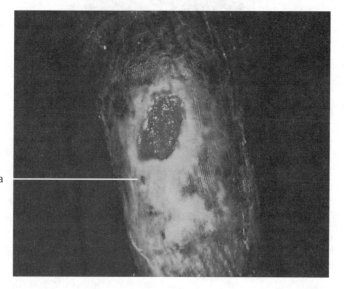

healed closed area

Figure 8–1 Full-Thickness Venous Stasis Ulcer on Dark-Skinned Person. Healed skin will remain light.

Clinical Objectives:
(1) Clean
(2) Keep moist
(3) Manage exudate
(4) Manage edema
See Color Plate 16.

Perforating Veins

- connect the deep and superficial veins
- contain valves to prevent backflow into superficial veins

Mechanisms of Venous Return

- calf muscle contraction (walking, etc.)
- variations in intra-abdominal and intrathoracic pressure
- venous valves, which allow unidirectional blood flow from superficial veins to deep veins

Venous Stasis Ulcers

A cascade of events occurs with venous disease, including increased hydrostatic pressure, venous hypertension, and venous stasis ulceration. In chronic venous

healed ulcer

ulcer, slough base

Figure 8–2 Venous Stasis Ulcer, Right Medial Ankle. Note edema, gaiter staining, and closed wound on left leg.

Clinical Objectives:
(1) Clean
(2) Keep moist
(3) Manage exudate
(4) Manage edema
See Color Plate 17.

Figure 8–3 Venous Stasis Ulcer. Shallow wound bed, irregular shape, wound bed ruddy red with some yellow slough.

Clinical Objectives:
(1) Clean
(2) Keep moist
(3) Manage exudate
(4) Manage edema
See Color Plate 18.

hypertension, damaged valves in the deep and perforating veins with backflow to superficial veins cause:

- dilation of veins
- edema
- increased pressure in the superficial veins
- further valve damage

Various theories as to the exact cause of the ulcerations are debated and include:

- the Fibrin Cuff Theory (Falanga, 1997, p. 166; Morison and Moffatt, 1997, p. 183)
- the White Cell Trapping Theory (Morison and Moffatt, 1997, p. 183)
- the Mechanical Theory (Falanga, 1997, pp. 166–168; Morison and Moffatt, 1997, p. 183)

ASSESSMENT

Predisposing Factors

- family history
- gender (higher incidence in women)
- pregnancy
- low-fiber diet
- obesity
- leg injury
- occupations that require standing
- smoking
- history of major leg trauma
- history of deep vein thrombosis (DVT)
- history of venous ligation or stripping

Clinical Signs

- brown/red staining of the skin in the gaiter area (hemosiderin staining)
- extremely dry, scaly skin or weepy, itchy, and erythematous skin (stasis eczema, dermatitis)
- peripheral edema that increases with prolonged standing and/or sitting (Prolonged edema gives the leg the appearance of an upside-down champagne bottle.)
- distention of tiny veins on medial aspect of the foot (ankle flare)
- induration of the tissue of lower leg (lipodermatosclerosis)
- thinning of the dermis
- history of an ulcer
- nonpitting ankle edema that doesn't resolve with elevation (woody fibrosis)

Ulcer (Typical Appearance)

- irregularly shaped wound (not typically round or with even wound edges)
- location on the medial aspect of the lower leg and ankle (common)
- painless (Patient may have a dull ache or heavy feeling particularly at night; unrelieved pain indicates further complicating factors.)
- extension into the dermal skin layer (frequent)
- ruddy red wound bed, with granular tissue; may have some yellow slough or yellow to brown fibrin
- exudate present (serous or serosanguineous)
- variable size

The etiology of the ulcer may not be known to the patient.

TREATMENT CHOICES

Goals

- reduce edema
- reduce blood pressure in the superficial venous system
- aid venous return to the heart
- utilize appropriate topical therapy to provide moist wound healing
- educate to prevent recurrence
- educate on importance of compression stockings after the ulcer has healed

Simple Diagnostics

- history and physical assessment
- Doppler ultrasonography: ankle-brachial index (ABI)

Further studies could include color-flow duplex imaging to help identify areas of valvular incompetence and/or photoplethysmography.

Compression Wraps (Exhibit 8–1)

The purpose of compression is to eliminate or reduce edema and to assist with venous return. Controversy exists over the amount of compression.

Effective compression must provide extraluminal pressure greater than intraluminal pressure (Rudolph, 1998, p. 251).

> **TIP** A lack A lack of wound improvement in 2 to 3 weeks is an indication for a complete reassessment of the patient.

Contraindications include arterial involvement as determined by diagnostics, deep vein thrombosis, cellulitis, severe leg deformity, and acute congestive heart failure.

Exhibit 8–1 Methods of Edema Management

Elimination and control of edema may be accomplished through leg elevation, exercise, and the use of compression therapy. A combination of the above-mentioned therapies is often necessary to achieve the desired control of edema in the affected limb(s). Clients should be encouraged to elevate their legs as often as possible and in general to avoid any length of time with their legs in a dependent position. Exercise that works the calf muscle pump while the client is using the appropriate compression garment or wrap should be encouraged. Clients may also find that elevation of the foot of the bed is helpful to facilitate leg elevation while sleeping. This is not useful for the client with heart disease, such as congestive heart failure. It is not unusual to find clients requesting a diuretic or water pill to facilitate the removal of the edema. The health care provider is encouraged to see this as an opportunity to provide client education about the futility of diuretics as a primary treatment for edema. Diuretics may be useful as an adjuvant therapy, especially if a sequential compression pump is to be used for the client with compromised cardiac function; however, diuretics are not a long-term solution to edema management. Appropriate for edema management are leg elevation and exercise, elastic wraps, tubular bandages, paste bandages, four-layer bandaging, graduated compression stockings, and intermittent sequential compression devices. A discussion of each follows.

LEG ELEVATION WITH EXERCISE

Leg elevation facilitates the removal of fluid through utilization of gravity to assist venous return. For leg elevation to be successful, the legs must be higher than the heart. Simply placing the feet on a stool is of no benefit. To facilitate leg elevation, the client may find it helpful to place one or two bricks under the foot end of the bed, which elevates the legs higher than the heart during sleep. It is helpful to demonstrate on the exam table or hospital bed by elevating the legs and then reclining on the surface. Clients should be encouraged to exercise the feet and ankles while elevating the legs. Stress that leg elevation can be intermittent and that total bed rest is not recommended. Intermittent leg elevation during the day for 20–30 minutes at a time for a total of at least two hours a day is a reasonable goal.

COMPRESSION THERAPY (ELASTIC AND TUBULAR BANDAGES)

Compression therapy works with exercise to facilitate the movement of excess fluid from the lower extremity. The level of compression needed for edema secondary to venous disease is approximately 40 mm Hg. For the client who is able to walk and work the calf muscles, 40 mm Hg compression is recommended. A client with dependent edema who is unable to work the calf muscles will not tolerate this level of compression, and a lower level of compression (Class 1 or Class 2) should be considered. (See Table 8–1, p. 142.) Elastic bandages are relatively easy to apply, inexpensive, and easily removed. As with all compression garments/devices, it is best to apply the bandages within 20 minutes of waking and placing the feet below the level of the heart. Most compression wraps giving at least Class 2 compression are removed at night. Bandages do require practice to apply correctly, and the skill needs to be taught to the client and caregiver. Manufacturer's guidelines should always be followed when applying the elastic bandage. The most common application technique is the spiral. Several types of bandages are now available with printed rectangles that when stretched to squares apply the correct level of compression. These markings facilitate correct wrapping of an extremity.

Tubular bandages provide light compression. One should be careful to select bandages that are tapered at the ankle. Straight tubular bandages provide compression that is higher at the calf than at the ankle. These are not as useful for the client with edema.

PASTE (UNNA BOOT) BANDAGES

Paste bandages such as the Unna boot are widely used in the treatment of leg ulcers and in the control of edema. The boot was developed in the 1880s by a German physician, Paul Gerson Unna, and consists of a fine gauze impregnated with zinc oxide, gelatin, and glycerin (some varieties also include calamine). The gauze is applied without tension in a circular fashion from the foot to just below the knee. Paste bandages do not provide compression; however, as the boot dries and stiffens, the leg cannot continue to swell. Application of a compression wrap over the boot will enhance compression and protect the client's clothing from the moist paste of the boot. A paste bandage is routinely changed every four to seven days.

FOUR-LAYER BANDAGING

An alternative to the paste bandage is the four-layer bandage developed at Charing Cross Hospital in London. The four-layer bandage provides graduated, sustained compression through the application of a series of layers, providing protection, padding, and compression. The dressing is removed weekly.

GRADUATED COMPRESSION STOCKINGS

Graduated compression stockings assist venous return, thereby reducing edema. The client should be measured and fitted for compression stockings when the edema is absent or minimal. These stockings are then applied before the client has gotten out of bed or at least within 20 minutes of rising. Stockings may be difficult to get on, and devices are available to assist in donning. A nonambulatory client does not need moderate or high compression and will likely better tolerate a lower-compression (18–24 mm Hg) stocking. Stockings do wear out and need to be replaced at the frequency recommended by the manufacturer. Many clients prefer to order two stockings (or two pairs) to prolong the life of the individual stocking and allow for laundering.

SEQUENTIAL COMPRESSION THERAPY

Sequential compression therapy has gained popularity for the management of lower extremity edema. The leg sleeve (either knee-high or thigh-high) is divided into 3-, 5-, and 10-chamber styles with peak pressures of 45 to 60 mm Hg at the ankle. The sleeve inflates first at the ankle, followed 2.5 seconds later at the calf chambers, and 3 seconds later at the thigh chambers. Each successive chamber inflates less, and the total inflation is sustained for approximately 5 seconds followed by complete deflation. The cycle repeats every 7–8 seconds for the prescribed treatment period, which may range from 1 to 2 hours twice per day. Clients should be encouraged to follow treatment with application of either a fitted stocking or a compression bandage to maintain edema control. Use of compression therapy at night while sleeping is not recommended. Clients with congestive heart disease should be monitored closely for tolerance of the intravascular fluid burden with compression therapy.

Source: Adapted from Wiersema-Bryant, L. A. (1998). Management of edema. In C. Sussman & B. M. Bates-Jensen (Eds.), *Wound care: A collaborative practice manual for physical therapists and nurses,* (2nd ed., pp. 180–198), Gaithersburg, MD: Aspen.

Types of Wraps

Follow the manufacturer's instructions. A few examples of different compression wraps are listed below. There are many more available.

- single-layer bandaging (e.g., Unna Boot™, Tubigrip™, Comprilan™)
- multilayer bandaging (e.g., Profore™, Unna-Flex™)
- graduated compression wraps (e.g., Profore™, SurePress™, Duoderm Sustained Compression Bandage™)
- compression wrap systems (e.g., CirAid™, Thera-Boot™, CircPlus™)
- mechanical graduated or sequential (lymphedema) pumps (e.g., Flow-press, Sof-Pres). Be sure to check the access in your area and the reimbursement of the pumps for the diagnosis of venous stasis ulcers.
- Treatment is usually performed one to two times per day for a specific amount of time.
- Pumps can be contraindicated for patients with congestive heart failure.

Local Wound Treatment

- Clean the wound with normal saline or a commercially prepared wound cleanser.
- Some compression wraps are impregnated with zinc oxide, gelatin, and glycerin pastes.

TIPS
- Change the first one or two compression wraps more frequently than the manufacturer of the compression wrap recommends. If the manufacturer suggests weekly changes, change it twice a week for the first one or two changes to assess the patient's tolerance to compression and the amount of wound exudate. The amount of exudate will drive your decision on the addition of an absorbent dressing under the compression such as a foam or alginate.
- Cleansing usually removes the odor that is present when the compression wrap is changed.
- Always provide the patient with the signs and symptoms of complications and what to do should they occur. Look for signs such as:
  - change in appearance of the toes—dusky or purple discoloration
  - increase in amount of discomfort or pain in the extremity
- Should either of the above occur, the patient should call the emergency number that you have provided for your agency and/or remove the compression wrap. When the edema begins to subside, many patients feel more comfortable with the wrap in place.
- Manage exudate with local wound treatment to prevent periwound maceration.
- Compress until the wound has healed to provide compliance and continuity.

- For highly exudating ulcers, use foams, alginates, and hydrofiber dressings under the compression wrap.
- Use hydrocolloid dressings under compression wraps when the wound is no longer highly exudative.
- Moisturize the leg and foot before applying compression.
- Measure the circumference of the leg to document the change in edema. Some measure 2, 6, and 8 inches above the ankle. This provides specific information on the effectiveness of a graduated compression wrap on the edema.
- Compression wraps are not all applied the same way. Some manufacturers recommend a spiral wrap while others recommend a figure eight. Follow the manufacturer's recommendations for the product you have selected to use. It is also wise to be taught how to wrap before attempting to apply a compression wrap to a patient.
- Should leg elevation be used, the leg should be elevated above the level of the heart to be effective.

EXPECTED OUTCOMES

- With compression, the wound will decrease dimensions quickly, sometimes with each dressing change.
- Without compression, long-term chronic wound management may be necessary due to the underlying pathology.

PREVENTION

Patient Education

- Explain the cause of ulcerations. Use a simple explanation of the difficulty the blood has in the return to the heart, including the function of support stockings/hosiery.
- Emphasize the importance of the long-term use of support stockings/compression hosiery (**Table 8–1**).
- Tell the patient to elevate legs above the level of the heart when sitting (**Exhibit 8–2**).
- Tell the patient to avoid crossing his or her legs.
- Stress exercise.
- Stress weight loss. A restriction of sodium intake is frequently beneficial.
- Counsel on smoking cessation.

See **Exhibit 8–3**.

Table 8–1 Vascular Support Options

Level of Support	Examples	Recommendations for Use
Light support (8–14 mm Hg)	Fashion hosiery Jobst Sigvarus	Edema prevention for persons engaged in activities/work that require standing/sitting without much activity; examples: beautician, cashier, factory worker, some nursing positions
Antiembolism stockings (16–18 mm Hg)	Anti-EM/GP (Jobst) TED stockings	Deep vein thrombosis prophylaxis Nonambulatory clients with edema
Low compression (18–24 mm Hg)	Relief (Jobst) Elastic wraps Paste bandage	Nonambulatory clients with edema Nonambulatory clients with edema failing 16–18 mm Hg stockings Clients with dependent edema
Low to moderate compression (25–35 mm Hg)	Fast-Fit (Jobst) Custom fit Double reverse elastic wrap Four-layer bandage	Edema secondary to venous insufficiency Edema in client able to participate in exercise rehab
Moderate compression (30–40 mm Hg)	Ultimate (Jobst) Custom stocking (Jobst, Sigvarus) Sequential pump Four-layer bandage (Profore, SurePress)	Edema with/without ulceration Edema that persists in spite of lower-level compression options Ulcer that failed to heal after 6 months
High compression (40–50 mm Hg)	Vairox (Jobst) Custom stockings (Jobst, Sigvarus) Sequential pump	Edema secondary to lymphedema

Note: Check with Medicare and private insurance about reimbursement for support hose.
Source: Adapted from Wiersema-Bryant, L. A. (1998). Management of edema. In C. Sussman & B. M. Bates-Jensen. (Eds.) *Wound care: A collaborative practice manual for physical therapists and nurses,* (2nd ed. p. 181.). Gaithersburg, MD: Aspen.

Exhibit 8–2 Patient Guide: Leg Elevation and Exercise

DEFINITION
Elevate the legs higher than the level of the heart, with or without foot and ankle exercise, to allow gravity to assist in the removal of fluid from the legs

ADVANTAGES
- no costs associated with the procedure
- effective when used regularly in combination with other form(s) of compression bandaging or stockings

- no special equipment required
- involves client in active participation in edema reduction

DISADVANTAGES

- Exercise/elevation requires consistent performance in order to be of benefit.
- Some people may be unable to elevate legs higher than the heart (e.g., clients with obesity, congestive heart failure, or orthopedic limitations).
- Sitting may not be allowed at work for leg elevation.
- Exercise/elevation may be ineffective in some forms of swelling.

EQUIPMENT NEEDED

- clean surface upon which to recline
- minute timer (optional)

FREQUENCY

Every 2–3 hours during the day for 20–30 minutes for a total of 2 or more hours per day

WHEN TO USE

When edema of the lower extremities occurs due to impaired venous return

WHEN *NOT* TO USE

- if you are very obese
- if you have hardening of the arteries (atherosclerosis) and pain with leg elevation
- if you have congestive heart failure and a limited ability to recline in a horizontal position
- if you have other medical conditions that limit your ability to recline in a horizontal position

PROCEDURE

1. Recline horizontally on a clean, comfortable surface (bed or recliner chair).
2. Elevate legs approximately 30 degrees so that feet are higher than the heart. Rest feet against wall or footboard of bed.
3. Set timer for 20 to 30 minutes (optional).
4. With one leg at a time, flex and extend foot against wall or footboard, then make circles (rotate) with the foot/ankle. Do 5–10 repetitions with each foot, then rest and repeat until timer goes off.
5. Remove and rewrap leg if compression bandage is being used.

EXPECTED RESULTS

Your swelling and pain/discomfort are relieved with leg elevation.

HELPFUL HINTS

- Use of a kitchen-type minute timer is helpful to ensure an adequate amount of time.
- Work up to 20–30 minutes gradually if it is too much when starting out.
- Be creative at work in looking for opportunities to exercise (walking, stair climbing, marching in place).

Source: Adapted from Wiersema-Bryant, L. A. (1998). Management of edema. In C. Sussman & B. M. Bates-Jensen (Eds.), *Wound care: A collaborative practice manual for physical therapists and nurses,* (2nd ed., pp. 185–186), Gaithersburg, MD: Aspen.

Exhibit 8–3 Patient Guide: Guidelines for Patients with Venous Insufficiency or Wounds

GIVE YOUR LEGS A REST

- Elevate your feet above your heart while sleeping and at regular times during the day (elevate foot of bed or mattress).
- Avoid work that requires you to stand or sit with your feet on the ground for long periods. Change positions frequently.
- Take walks to help leg muscles "pump" fluids into your legs.

GIVE YOUR LEGS SUPPORT

- Wear professionally made support stockings that apply pressure from ankle to knee or other compression devices. (Your physician can help you choose the kind that is right for you and send you to a professional who will properly measure your legs for stocking size.)
- Have at least two pairs of support stockings available so you can change them daily. After laundering, hang them up to dry. Do not put them in a dryer.
- Always put on support stockings early in the morning before fluid pools in lower legs.
- Wear support stockings all day and then remove them in the evening when going to sleep.
- Buy new stockings every 6 months so their strength doesn't wear out.
- Avoid ACE® bandages. It is extremely difficult to wrap them properly to provide the pressure you need.
- If your physician has prescribed the use of a compression pump, follow the instructions completely. It may take a little time to adjust to the pumping procedure.

TAKE CARE OF YOUR SKIN

- Wash your lower legs and feet regularly with mild soap and water.
- Use moisturizing creams and emollients after washing. Don't put lotion on the wounds. It is important not to use petroleum or lanolin-based creams when wearing stockings that contain latex. Your physician or pharmacist may suggest appropriate brands.
- Be particularly careful to avoid activities that are likely to cause injury to legs or feet. *Prevention is very important.*

WATCH FOR SKIN CHANGES

Pay particular attention to signs of progressive venous insufficiency:

- **swelling** that does not go away quickly when you lie down
- **discoloration,** especially brownish skin discoloration around ankles and lower legs
- **dryness and/or itching** in the same areas
- **any wound or bruise** that doesn't go away within a week

IF YOU HAVE A WOUND

- Keep it clean. Keep minor wounds clean and protect with a bandage.
- Avoid strong antiseptics. Many antiseptics such as hydrogen peroxide, povidone–iodine, and sodium hypochlorite can damage skin and interfere with healing.
- Always wear support stockings during your daily activities. If it is difficult to wear them over the bandage, put on a knee-length nylon stocking first and wear the support stocking over it.

- Watch the wound carefully. You will need to describe any changes to your physician. Remember that any wound may turn into a chronic wound, and early treatment has been shown to be beneficial.

IF YOUR WOUND DOESN'T HEAL IN 1 WEEK

Don't put off seeing your physician. *Any wound that doesn't heal in a week should be seen by your physician.*

REMEMBER

- You are a vital part of your treatment program, and it is essential that you faithfully follow all medical directions.
- Always consult your health care professional before making any change to your health care routine, if you have questions, or if your symptoms become worse.

Source: Courtesy of Curative Health Service, Hauppage, New York.

CASE STUDY

Mrs. Jan Evens, 66 years old, lives with her husband in a one-story home in a small Midwestern community. She has three adult children living nearby. Jan weighs 170 pounds and is 5 feet 5 inches tall. She has been a smoker, although she hasn't smoked in the last 10 years and has recently retired from a packaging company where she worked for the past 15 years, standing on an assembly line. Jan is not a diabetic.

Jan has been admitted to home care following surgery for a ruptured diverticular abscess and a colostomy. She has an open abdominal incision requiring a skilled nurse visit and has a long-standing lower leg ulcer. The physician's orders for the skilled nursing visit included not only care of the abdominal incision and colostomy teaching, but also ulcer care. Jan told her home care nurse she has had the ulcer for several years, and it has always embarrassed her. She usually wore slacks to hide it even during the summer. In the past, Jan treated the ulcer with various creams and antibiotic ointments and a bandage. It would get smaller, but it never healed completely.

An assessment of her lower leg reveals a moderate amount of edema of her lower leg and foot. Jan states that she had noticed that if she elevated her leg at night when she watched television, the swelling decreased. She does not have any leg pain. There is red/brown discoloration of the skin above her ankle (hemosiderin staining), prominent superficial leg veins, distention of the veins on the medial aspect of the foot (ankle flare), a hardened, indurated texture to the skin (lipodermatosclerosis), and dry, flaky skin (stasis dermatitis). The ulcer is a full-thickness wound on the medial aspect of the lower leg, measuring 6.0 cm long by 4.0 cm wide and approximately 1.0 cm deep. The wound edges are irregular and have a white discoloration (maceration from wound exudate). The wound bed is approximately 75% red, granular tissue and 25% yellow, fibrinous slough. The gauze dressing, applied the day before, is saturated with tannish colored drainage. The wound has no odor. An ABI, done in the home, is 0.8. A full report of the assessment findings including the ABI was telephoned to the physician.

A foam dressing was chosen to cover the wound. A hydrocolloid, alginate, or hydrofiber would also be appropriate; however, in this case, a foam was chosen to absorb the wound exudate evidenced by the maceration at the wound edges. In addition, a compression wrap was applied after obtaining a measurement of the leg circumference 2, 6, and 10 inches above the ankle. The measurements provided a reference point for the expected decrease in the edema with the use of compression. The first wrap was changed in 4 days to assess the wound and the patient's tolerance of compression. The patient was instructed to call if there was pain or blue/purple discoloration of the toes. Jan tolerated compression well, and the foam dressing adequately absorbed the wound exudate. The compression wrap was changed weekly thereafter. The wound was completely healed in less than 6 months. The patient wore light compression hosiery after healing. Light compression was selected to reduce recurrence and increase compliance. Dietary instructions, including methods to increase fiber and lower weight, were given to Jan. A light exercise program of walking was initiated to help with weight control and to increase the pumping action of the calf muscle, thereby assisting with venous return to the heart. Understanding the underlying cause of the ulceration, weight loss, regular exercise, and light compression were key elements in a prevention program for Jan.

REFERENCES

Falanga, V. (1997). Venous ulceration: Assessment, classification and management. In D. Krasner & D. Kane (Eds.), *Chronic wound care: A clinical source book for healthcare professionals* (2d ed., pp. 165–171). Wayne, PA: Health Management Publications.

Morison, M., & Moffatt, C. (1997). Leg ulcers. In M. Morison et al. (Eds.), *Nursing management of chronic wounds* (2d ed., pp. 177–220). Philadelphia, PA: Mosby.

Rudolph, D. (1998). Pathophysiology and management of venous ulcers. *Journal of Wound, Ostomy, and Continence Nursing, 25*(5), 248–255.

BIBLIOGRAPHY

Columbia University Medical Center. (2011). Wound healing: Treatment protocols, venous ulcer. Retrieved from http://www.columbiasurgery.org/cli/wound/venous_ulcer.html

Doughty, D. B., & Holbrook, R. (2007). Lower-extremity ulcers of vascular etiology. In R. A. Bryant & D. P. Nix, *Acute and chronic wounds: Current management concepts* (3rd ed., pp. 258–268, 277–304). St. Louis, MO. Mosby Elsevier.

Kunimoto, B. T. (2001). Management and prevention of venous leg ulcers: A literature-guided approach. *Ostomy Wound Management, 47*(6), 36–49.

Kunimoto, B. T., Casling, M., Gulliner, W., Houghton, P. Orstead, H., & Sibbold, R. G. (2001). Best practice for prevention and treatment of venous leg ulcers. *Ostomy Wound Management, 47*(2), 34–50.

Siegel, A. (1998). Noninvasive vascular testing. In C. Sussman & B. M. Bates-Jensen (Eds.), *Wound care: A collaborative practice manual for physical therapists and nurses* (pp. 127–135). Gaithersburg, MD: Aspen.

Sieggreen, M. Y., & Kline, R. A. (2000). Vascular ulcers. In S. Baranoski & E. A. Ayello (Eds.), *Wound care essentials: Practice principles* (pp. 271–310). Philadelphia, PA: Lippincott Williams & Wilkins.

Lower Leg Ulcers with Mixed Disease

Julie Phelps Maloy

It is not uncommon to be asked to evaluate and recommend treatment for an ulcer on the lower leg that clinically resembles a venous stasis ulcer but, after a complete assessment, is also shown to have arterial involvement (**Figure 9–1**; **Color Plate 19**). This patient has mixed disease or venous stasis disease with underlying arterial involvement. This means not only are there incompetent valves in the veins creating difficulty with the venous return, but also probable atherosclerosis in the arteries restricting the blood flow into the extremity. The patient may or may not also be a diabetic. Compression is the treatment of choice for venous stasis ulcers, however, only if there is adequate blood supply to the extremity evidenced by vascular studies. If you jump to a conclusion that the ulcer is a venous stasis ulcer based on a visual assessment, you could compress a patient who is not a candidate for compression, further restricting the blood flow to the extremity and hastening an amputation. Some have estimated that as many as 21% of patients with lower leg ulcers have an arterial component (Morison & Moffatt, 1997, p. 186). It is extremely important to know the etiology of the ulcers for which you recommend treatments.

ETIOLOGY

Chronic venous stasis ulcers are caused by damaged valves in the deep and perforating veins, with backflow to superficial veins causing:

- dilation of veins
- edema
- increased pressure in the superficial veins
- further valve damage

Arterial ulcers are caused by a lack of blood supply with the most common cause being atherosclerosis.

Figure 9–1 Ulcer with Mixed Disease. Patient is not a surgical candidate.
Clinical Objectives:
(1) Prevent infection
(2) Provide protection
(3) Absorb exudate
See Color Plate 19.

ASSESSMENT

Risk Factors

- hypertension
- smoking
- diabetes
- hyperlipidemia
- obesity
- family history
- occupations requiring standing

Clinical Signs

Lower Leg

- brown staining of the skin (hemosiderin staining)
- dry, scaly skin (stasis eczema)
- peripheral edema (can be only slight)

- thinning of the dermis
- induration of the tissue of the lower leg (lipodermatosclerosis)
- distention of the tiny veins on the medial aspect of the foot (ankle flare)
- pulses palpable or not palpable in the dorsalis pedis and posterior tibialis
- possible accompanying cellulitis
- possible thickened, yellow, fragile toenails

Ulcer

- irregularly shaped or rounded wound edges
- located on the medial, front, or lateral aspect of the lower leg or ankle
- pain, cramping, or burning (can be masked if the patient is a diabetic)
- pale or ruddy and granular wound bed
- exudate (usually present)
- etiology due to trauma or unknown by the patient
- long-standing duration
- slough or dry eschar in the wound bed

Complications

- wound infection
- gangrene (black or brown necrotic tissue caused by a lack of blood supply, frequently at the most distal aspects of the leg and foot; if toe is affected, can wither into a hard mass and separate by autolysis)
- amputation

TREATMENT CHOICES

Goals

Goals are dependent upon the physical condition of the patient.

- Establish adequate circulation to the affected area when the patient is a surgical candidate.
- After establishing adequate circulation surgically,
  - Reduce the edema.
  - Utilize appropriate topical therapy.
- For the nonsurgical candidate,
  - Utilize appropriate topical therapy.
  - Do not include compression therapy. Compression therapy further restricts the compromised arterial blood flow to the leg.

Diagnostics

- history and physical assessment
- noninvasive studies of the arterial system using a Doppler ultrasound to determine the ankle-brachial index (ABI)
  - A normal ABI is considered to be 0.9–1.1.
  - Claudication can occur between 0.5 and 0.6.
  - Tissue loss and rest pain (signaling a threatened limb) can occur at < 0.5.
    Most consider an ABI to be invalid in a diabetic patient. The increased atherosclerosis with resulting calcified vessels causes a falsely elevated ABI.
- further vascular evaluation

Surgical Intervention for Revascularization

See bibliography for resources containing further surgical information.

Medical Management

Nonsurgical candidates require good wound care and patient education. Nurses need to be aware that without restoring an adequate blood supply, this is usually a nonhealing wound that can get progressively worse.

Local Wound Management

- Clean the wound with normal saline or a commercially prepared wound cleanser.
- Utilize wound dressings that provide a moist wound environment, preventing the wound from drying out. A dry wound causes increased cell death and necrosis. Note: The current thought is that heels and toes are an exception to the moist wound dressings rule: If heels and toes are covered with hard, black eschar, leave them covered with the black eschar unless there are signs and symptoms of infection, leakage of exudate, or odor. Removing eschar that has no other symptoms increases the opportunity for infection and can quickly lead to an amputation due to the already compromised blood supply to the area.
- Select a dressing that meets the needs of the wound.

PREVENTION

Patient Education

- Explain the underlying cause of the ulceration(s).
- Discuss blood glucose control with the diabetic patient.

> **TIP** Even though this ulcer can strongly resemble a venous stasis ulcer, don't treat it using compression if an ABI indicates this is a threatened limb. Compression is not an option for all patients with lower leg ulcers and edema.

- Counsel on cessation of smoking.
- Stress weight control and a mild exercise program both for weight control and to build collateral circulation if the patient is able to tolerate this without intermittent claudication. Explain the benefits of a low-fat diet.
- Discuss blood pressure management (including stress reduction classes, if appropriate).
- Include pharmacologic education of drug interactions and reactions for patients on medication.
- Explain signs and symptoms of complications along with what to do should they occur:
  - Look for deepening of the ulcer along with increasing amounts of exudate, erythema, streaks of red running up the leg, pain, and/or the presence of black tissue (eschar or gangrene).
  - Call the physician, or if there is an emergent situation, go to the emergency department.

CASE STUDY

Randy Rudicle was referred to your agency following discharge from the hospital. He had been admitted to the hospital because his recently diagnosed diabetes mellitus was poorly controlled. His medical history includes coronary heart disease and diabetes, which he had attempted to control by dietary measures. He had angioplasty with stent placement in two coronary arteries 6 months earlier. He required home care follow-up for his recently diagnosed diabetes mellitus, which now requires the use of insulin. He also requires a skilled nurse for treatment of a long-standing ulcer on his right lower leg. Randy is 66 years old, 6 feet tall, and 270 pounds. He has been a two-pack-a-day cigarette smoker, although he had stopped smoking 6 months ago when his coronary artery disease was diagnosed. He is retired; however, he had worked in an industrial environment on an assembly line most of his working years. In addition to his other medical conditions, Randy has an ulcer on the front of his lower right leg. He fell down a few steps of a ladder when he was painting the trim on his house and skinned the front of his leg a year ago. He has tried several home remedies and, to his frustration, the ulcer has increased in size. Randy's leg has a small amount of edema, which is unilateral. The right lower leg has some hemosiderin staining extending beyond the ulcer approximately 4.0 cm. There is not any induration. The gauze 4×4 dressing, which was applied in the early morning, is saturated with tan drainage. There is no odor. The ulcer, measuring 5.0 cm long by 3.0 cm wide, is oval in shape with even wound edges. The wound bed has a ruddy granular appearance. The ulcer is now a full-thickness ulcer. The ulcer has many of the clinical signs of a venous stasis ulcer; however, due to Randy's diagnosis of diabetes, an ABI is not a reliable test to determine arterial involvement. A referral from the physician for a vascular evaluation at a vascular laboratory will be necessary before a complete treatment plan for the wound can be identified. The testing reveals arterial involvement requiring revascularization. Randy does not want any further surgical procedures at this time. He is overwhelmed with all of his recent medical problems. His choice is for a more conservative path for wound care.

The care of this patient and the long-term management are complex. It will be necessary to follow up on and reinforce the diabetes education that began in the hospital, including dietary reinforcement, the correct administration of insulin, blood glucose monitoring, proper foot care, and the potential for slow-healing wounds. In addition, any further education on coronary heart disease could be indicated along with providing support for Randy's progress on smoking cessation and stress management. A light exercise program to help with weight control and to decrease stress would be ideal when Randy is no longer homebound; however, with the complication of arterial disease in his extremities, he could experience intermittent claudication from a decrease of oxygen to the muscles. It will be necessary for the nurse to educate Randy on good wound care utilizing the principles of moist wound healing. The signs and symptoms of wound complications requiring a call to his physician should also be included. The probability of wound healing is minimal in a wound that has the complication of significant arterial disease. The dressing selection should include one that will provide moist wound healing, absorb the exudate, protect the wound from further trauma, and be manageable and affordable for Randy and his wife. This could include a foam, alginate, hydrofiber, or composite dressing. Not all wounds have an outcome that nurses have come to expect. Randy's decision could be the best for him at the present. He could have difficulty in healing after revascularization until his diabetes is in better long-term control. Either way, an amputation could occur in his future.

REFERENCE

Morison, M., & Moffatt, C. (1997). Leg ulcers. In M. Morison, et al. (Eds.), *Nursing management of chronic wounds* (2d ed., pp. 177–220). Philadelphia, PA: Mosby.

BIBLIOGRAPHY

Doughty, D. B., & Holbrook, R. (2007). Lower-extremity ulcers of vascular etiology. In R. A. Bryant & D. P. Nix (Eds.), *Acute and chronic wounds: Current management concepts* (3rd ed., pp. 258–306). St. Louis, MO. Mosby Elsevier.

Mosquera, D. (2011). Chronic venous insufficiency and leg ulceration. D. Mosquera, Ltd. Retrieved October 17, 2011 from http://www.vascular.co.nz/chronic_venous_insufficiency%20and%20leg%20ulceration.htm#What causes leg ulcers.

O'Brien, S. P., et al. (1998). Epidemiology, risk factors, and management of peripheral vascular disease. *Ostomy/Wound Management, 44*(9), 68–75.

Siegel, A. (1998). Noninvasive vascular testing. In C. Sussman & B. M. Bates-Jensen (Eds.), *Wound care: A collaborative practice manual for physical therapists and nurses* (pp. 127–135). Gaithersburg, MD: Aspen.

Diabetic Neuropathic Foot Ulcers

Julie Phelps Maloy

Diabetes is a complicated chronic disease. The information presented here is not meant to oversimplify diabetes. A high blood glucose can contribute to many complications. One set of complications is the diabetic neuropathic foot ulcer. A person with diabetes can have venous stasis or arterial ulcers; however, when the reference is made to a diabetic ulcer, it is most commonly considered to be a neuropathic ulcer located on the plantar surface of the foot. Foot ulcers are the most common cause of hospitalization among those with diabetes. Over one-half of the lower limb amputations are performed on diabetic patients. Eighty-five percent of diabetes-related amputations are preceded by a foot ulcer (Armstrong, et al., 1998, p. 123; Kravitz, McGuire, and Shanahan, 2003, p. 69). Research has shown that the amputation of one toe is enough to contribute to the development of deformities of the remaining toes and to the formation of a new ulcer on the same foot as well as the other (contralateral) foot (Levin, 1998, pp. 129–130). Many factors contribute to the foot ulcer, including lack of sensation; bone and muscle changes resulting in toe, ankle, and foot deformities; lack of perspiration; friction; and callus buildup. Diabetics have impaired wound healing ability. Once the ulceration occurs, the problem is compounded. If the wound is not aggressively treated, infection quickly occurs, leading to gangrene and an amputation. This sets the stage for further amputations, and the cycle continues.

ETIOLOGY

Many factors contribute to diabetic neuropathic foot ulcers. These factors usually include sensory, motor, and autonomic neuropathy. These conditions are not reversible and will continue to worsen over time.

Background

An increased blood glucose interferes with the structural integrity of collagen, enzymatic reactions, and the functions of the cell membrane. (More in-depth information on diabetes and wound healing is found in Levin, et al., 1993; Mulder, 2000; Steed, 1997, pp. 172–177.)

Peripheral Neuropathy

Motor

- toe changes (claw toes/hammer toes)
- thinning of the fat pad over the ball of the foot (metatarsal head)
- atrophy of the muscles (interosseous) of the metatarsals

Sensory

- loss of sensation

Autonomic Neuropathy

- increased blood flow leads to increased bone reabsorption, which can cause joint collapse and Charcot foot
- decreased perspiration leads to dry, cracked skin

Peripheral Vascular Disease

- impaired wound healing
- atherosclerosis (occurs at a younger age and advances more rapidly in the person with diabetes)
- cholesterol emboli

Summary

- Lower leg has shiny skin, dependent rubor, hair loss, subcutaneous fat atrophy, and delayed superficial plexus filling time.
- Atherosclerosis of the vessels in the leg leads to a decrease in blood flow to the leg and foot and therefore a decrease of oxygen and nutrition to the extremity.
- A decrease in touch sensation, temperature sensation, and pain perception creates an inability to feel any discomfort with the shoes or any trauma to the feet.
- A lack of perspiration creates dry feet that crack, providing a hiding place for bacteria and a potential for infection.
- Deterioration of the muscles results in changes in the toes, causing a change in the weight distribution through the forefoot.
- Deterioration of the bones in the foot (Charcot foot) leads to deformities and changes in the weight distribution of the foot.
- Sliding of the foot causes friction and callus buildup. If a cavity forms under the callus, an ulcer is formed. Dry cracked skin and the bacteria contained there empty bacteria into the ulcer bed, leading to infection, gangrene, and possibly amputation.

CHARCOT FOOT

See **Figures 10–1** and **10–2**; **Color Plate 20**.

Stages of Development (Levin, 1998, p. 132)

First Stage (Acute Stage)

- Usually there has been some type of trauma to the foot or ankle.
- The clinical picture is hot, red, swollen, with bounding pulses, resembling a cellulitis.
- Treatment is nonweight bearing, which continues until the skin temperature returns to normal. A total contact case is often used.

Second Stage

- This stage occurs because the patient ambulated in the first stage.
- The foot develops fragmentation (pieces of bone break off) and fractures.
- The toes take on a pointed appearance.
- Changes can develop as early as 2 to 3 weeks after stage 1.

Figure 10–1 Classic Charcot Rocker-Bottom Foot Deformity.

Figure 10–2 Neuropathic Ulcer; Charcot Foot.
Clinical Objectives:
(1) Off-loading techniques
(2) Manage infection if present
(3) Manage exudate
See Color Plate 20.

Third Stage

- The foot is deformed due to the collapse of the joints in stage 2.
- The clinical picture is a rocker-bottom/clubfoot look due to the collapse of the plantar arch.

Fourth Stage

- Should the patient continue to walk on the foot, unprotected ulceration develops due to the shift of pressure.
- Ulceration quickly leads to infection, gangrene, and eventual amputation.

ASSESSMENT

Risk Factors (Elftman, 1998, pp. 315–345; Kravitz, McGuire, & Shanahan, 2003, p. 69)

- poor glycemic control
- loss of sensation of the feet

- decreased perspiration
- lack of attention to the feet and nails
- previous history of ulceration
- structural deformity
- limited joint range of motion
- obesity
- diabetes of 15 years or longer
- smoking
- alcohol use

Clinical Signs

- callus buildup on the plantar surface of the foot (also referred to as a "hot spot") (**Figures 10–3** and **10–4**; **Color Plates 21** and **22**)
- ulceration over the metatarsal heads or the plantar surface of the hallux (heel)
- ulceration on the plantar surface of foot deformity (often with a punched-out appearance)
- cracks in the skin between the toes or at the base of the toes on the plantar surface of the foot

Figure 10–3 Diabetic Ulcer Needs Saucer-Style Debridement of Callus. Note dry skin at ankle, typical of diabetics.

Clinical Objectives:
(1) Clean
(2) Keep moist
See Color Plate 21.
(3) Manage exudate
(4) Eliminate pressure (nonweight bearing)

Figure 10–4 Diabetic Foot Ulcer with Hypergranulation Tissue, Callus Margin.

Clinical Objectives:

(1) Clean   (3) Manage exudate

(2) Keep moist   (4) Eliminate pressure

See Color Plate 22.

Ulcer

Assess the ulcer for:

- location
- length, width, and depth
  - The NPUAP staging system for pressure ulcers can be used.
  - Wagner scale for diabetic foot ulcers (**Exhibit 10–1**).
  - partial thickness and full thickness
- exudate (color and amount)
- erythema (around the ulcer)
- edema (in the tissue around the ulcer)
- wound bed (percentage of the wound bed with granulation, yellow devitalized tissue, and black eschar)
- odor
- suspected or confirmed infection
- undermining
- length of time the patient has had the ulcer

Check the foot for loss of protective sensation (**Exhibit 10–2**).

- presence or absence of pulses (dorsalis pedis, posterior tibialis)
- location of deformities
- condition of the toes and nails (who trims the nails and how)

Exhibit 10–1 Wagner Scale

Grade	Description
Grade 0	Skin intact
Grade 1	Superficial ulcer
Grade 2	Deeper ulcer to tendon or bone
Grade 3	Ulcer has abscess or osteomyelitis
Grade 4	Gangrene on forefoot
Grade 5	Gangrene over major portion of foot

Source: Reprinted with permission from F. E. W. Wagner, the Wagner Scale from *The dysvascular foot: A system for diagnosis and treatment, foot and ankle*, (Vol. 2, pp. 64–122), © 1981, Williams & Wilkins.

- condition of the skin, including the presence and locations of calluses, cracks, and fissures
- sensory examination using a Semmes-Weinstein monofilament
  - The patient should be supine or sitting with feet supported.
  - The patient should be able to identify the area on the plantar surface of the foot being touched with the monofilament.
- type of footwear used and how long the patient has been wearing the current shoes
- who inspects the feet for the patient and how often
- history of previous foot ulcerations/amputations

Complications

- deepening of the ulcer to the tendons and bone
- infection
  - Signs include increased amounts of drainage, erythema, pain, temperature, foul odor, and red streaks running up the leg from the ulcer.
  - This is a common complication that progresses to gangrene.
  - The best management depends on an early diagnosis, appropriate antibiotic therapy, and surgical debridement.
- gangrene
- amputation

TREATMENT CHOICES

Management of the Ulcer

- radiographic imaging to rule out osteomyelitis, foreign objects, and asymptomatic fractures
- debridement to remove necrotic tissue and determine the ulcer depth

Exhibit 10–2 Management of the Insensitive Foot in Diabetes

DIABETIC FOOT SCREEN	Date: _____
Patient's Name (Last, First, Middle) _____	ID No.:_____

Fill in the following blanks with an "R," "L," or "B" to indicate positive findings on the right, left, or both feet.

Has there been a change in the foot since last evaluation?   Yes ___   No ___

Is there a foot ulcer now or history of foot ulcer?   Yes ___   No ___

Does the foot have an abnormal shape?   Yes ___   No ___

Is there weakness in the ankle or foot?   Yes ___   No ___

Are the nails thick, too long, or ingrown?   Yes ___   No ___

Label sensory level with a "+" in the circled areas of the foot if the patient can feel the 10-gram (5.07 Semmes-Weinstein) nylon filament and "–" if he/she cannot feel the 10-gram filament.

RIGHT   LEFT

Label skin condition with
R—Redness,
S—Swelling,
W—Warmth,
D—Dryness,
M—Maceration

Callus ▨ Preulcer ▨ Ulcer ■ (note width/depth in cm)

Vascular:	Brachial Systolic Pressure	R_____	L_____
	Ankle Systolic Pressure	R_____	L_____
	Ischemic Index	R_____	L_____

Does the patient use footwear appropriate for his/her category?   Yes___   No___

RISK CATEGORY:

_____ 0 No loss of protective sensation.

_____ 1 Loss of protective sensation with no weakness, deformity, callus, preulcer, or history of ulceration.

_____ 2 Loss of protective sensation with weakness, deformity, preulcer, or callus, but no history of ulceration; or Ischemic Index < 0.45.

_____ 3 History of plantar ulceration.

Source: Reprinted with permission from J. C. Duffy & C. A. Payout, Figure 1 of Management of the Insensitive Foot in Diabetes, Military Medicine: *International Journal of AMSUS*, Vol. 155, No. 12, p. 575 © 1990, Association of Military Surgeons of the United States, The Society of the Federal Health Agencies.

- revascularization for those with limb-threatening arterial insufficiency
- biopsy for ulcers in an uncommon location
- aggressive antibiotic coverage when infection is present (Most common pathogens are aerobic, gram-positive staphylococci and streptococci, although other pathogens can be present, including anaerobes.)
- avoidance of weight bearing (Walking on the ulcer can cause further necrosis, delay healing, and force bacteria into deeper tissues. The best method is considered to be the total-contact cast—contraindicated for foot ulcers with abscess, osteomyelitis, or a similar deep infection or gangrene.)
- adequate nutrition including vitamins, minerals, protein, and good glucose control
- topical dressing chosen according to the location, size, depth, amount of drainage, and type of wound (The selection of a topical dressing without including the other items listed increases the probability of an amputation.)

PREVENTION

Management of Healed Ulcers

- Prevention of friction and callus buildup requires proper orthotics/ therapeutic footwear.
  - Those with Charcot foot need a molded shoe.
  - Podiatrists and/or certified pedorthists are qualified for the proper fitting of therapeutic shoes and insoles.
- Those with peripheral neuropathy, peripheral arterial disease, previous ulceration, or deformed feet are discouraged from jogging, prolonged walking, and treadmill exercises.
- Daily foot inspection by the patient or caregiver is vital.

Patient Education

- importance of foot care (**Exhibit 10–3**)
- control of blood sugar

TIP Medicare Part B and some medical insurance plans may pay a portion of the cost for therapeutic footwear for people with diabetes. Certain restrictions apply. Check with your insurance provider to find out if this is available for you.

NAIL CARE

- The goal depends upon the patient, but it generally includes improving comfort, reducing embarrassment from unattractive nails, and making the shoes less painful.

Exhibit 10–3 Patient Guide: Care of the Diabetic Foot

- Do not smoke.

- Inspect the feet daily for blisters, cuts, and scratches. The use of a mirror can aid in seeing the bottom of the feet. Always check between the toes.

- Wash feet daily. Dry carefully, especially between the toes.

- Avoid extremes of temperatures. Test water with hand, elbow, or thermometer before bathing.

- If feet feel cold at night, wear socks. Do not apply hot water bottles or heating pads. Do not use an electric blanket. Do not soak feet in hot water.

- Do not walk on hot surfaces, such as sandy beaches or on cement around swimming pools.

- Do not walk barefoot.

- Do not use chemical agents for removal of corns and calluses, corn plasters, or strong antiseptic solutions.

- Do not use adhesive tape on the feet.

- Inspect the inside of shoes daily for foreign objects, nail points, torn linings, and rough areas.

- If your vision is impaired, have a family member inspect your feet daily, trim nails, and buff calluses.

- For dry feet, use a very thin coat of a lubricating oil or cream. Apply this after bathing and drying feet. Do not put the oil or cream between the toes. Consult your physician for detailed instructions.

- Stockings: Wear properly fitting stockings. Do not wear mended stockings or stockings with seams. Change stockings daily.

- Do not wear garters.

- Shoes should be comfortable at the time of purchase. Do not depend on them to stretch out. Shoes should be made of leather. Purchase shoes late in the afternoon when feet are the largest. Running or special walking shoes may be worn after checking with your physician. Purchase shoes from shoe sales people who understand diabetic foot problems.

- Do not wear shoes without stockings.

- Do not wear sandals with thongs between the toes.

- In wintertime, take special precautions. Wear wool socks and protective foot gear such as fleece-lined boots.

- Cut nails straight across.

- Do not cut corns and calluses: follow instructions from your physician or podiatrist.

- Avoid crossing your legs; this can cause pressure on the nerves.

- See your physician regularly, and be sure that your feet are examined at each visit.

- Notify your physician or podiatrist at once should you develop a blister or sore on your feet.

- Be sure to inform your podiatrist that you are a diabetic.

Source: Reprinted with permission from J. C. Duffy and C. A. Payout, Figure 1 of Management of the Insensitive Foot in Diabetes, *Military Medicine: International Journal of AMSUS*, Vol. 155, No. 12, p. 575 © 1990, Association of Military Surgeons of the United States. The Society of the Federal Health Agencies.

- Instructions on proper assessment and trimming are needed because trimming dystrophic nails is considered to be debridement.
- Controversy exists in the literature on the best method of debriding nails. The overall result should be a smooth nail border without sharp edges in the corners.
- The nurse must always remember to wear gloves and a mask, and in some cases a gown, for protection from contaminants that are harbored under the nails and become airborne.
- Interventions include the following (Kelechi & Lukas, 1999, p. 53):
  - Assess overall hygiene, circulation, sensation, skin, toenails, mobility, condition of the footwear, and level of patient understanding.
  - Trimming nails includes the appropriate tools—a spring barrel nail nipper and emery board or pumice stone.
  - Basic foot care includes washing and drying the feet and applying an emollient; however, emollients should not be placed between the toes.
  - Corns, calluses, and dystrophic nails should be cared for by a nurse who has been taught nail debridement or by a physician or podiatrist.

TIP

- Even though it may look as though there is not an ulcer under a callus, it needs to be evaluated by an expert in your community (e.g., podiatrist, diabetic foot specialist).

- An ulcer that appears shallow can extend deep into the tissues of the foot.

- This is not the type of ulcer on which to try first one type of dressing and then another, thinking you will find a magical fix by the appropriate choice of a topical treatment. This ulcer needs aggressive treatment by someone who routinely treats diabetic foot ulcers.

- Lawsuits commonly result from amputations; providing appropriate care and referral is essential.

CASE STUDY

Joseph Alexander, who is 66 years old, obese, and a smoker, was referred to your agency from the Centerville Hospital following a brief hospitalization for poor blood glucose control and a foot infection. He had stepped on an unknown object and developed an ulcer on his left foot. While in the hospital, he received diabetic dietary instruction, and he was placed on intravenous antibiotic therapy for the infection that had resulted from the injury. He was discharged on oral antibiotics. Joseph, an insulin-dependent diabetic for 20 years, had developed peripheral neuropathy and was unaware when or how he injured his foot. He noticed blood on his sock, put a bandage on the spot, and had forgotten about it. When he had his feet up one evening watching television, his wife noticed the redness that was developing on the bottom (plantar surface) of his foot. She insisted that he see the physician, which had resulted in his hospitalization. During the admission interview, you discover that Joseph has no understanding of regular foot checks or of diabetic foot care. He purchases his shoes at the local discount store, but he tells you they have never been uncomfortable (remember he has peripheral neuropathy).

When you examine Joseph's feet, you discover a callus on the first metatarsal head (bottom of the foot below the great toe, commonly referred to as the ball of the foot) on the right foot. There is no discoloration, erythema, or exudate from the area. His toes on both feet are beginning to have a cocked-up appearance. His toenails on both feet are jagged, thick, and yellowed. Joseph tells you his feet are becoming flat although you do not see any erythema or swelling at the arch of either of his feet. They are not hot to the touch, which is a symptom of stage 1 in the development of acute Charcot inflammation. You are able to palpate pulses in both feet. The ulcer on the left foot is located on the heel (hallux) of his foot. The wound base is 80% yellow, devitalized tissue, and 20% granulation. There is 1.0 cm of erythema surrounding the 2.0 cm long × 1.5 cm wide ulcer. You are unable to tell the true depth of the ulcer due to the presence of the devitalized tissue; however, it is currently 0.5 cm deep. There is no odor, and the alginate dressing that was applied the day before is saturated with sanguineous exudate.

When you are presented with this or a similar case, there are a multitude of issues to address. Remember when you are putting these issues in priority order that not all physicians are diabetic specialists or understand the complexities of the diabetic foot. Who, in your area, are your referral sources for care of the diabetic foot ulcer, nail care, and footwear? Joseph has had a course of intravenous antibiotics, but not aggressive treatment of the ulcer. One short course of antibiotics is not the only treatment for this patient nor is a topical dressing that provides autolytic debridement. Infection is a common and quick complication, and the ulcer needs aggressive debridement, X-rays to see if there is osteomyelitis present, and off-loading of the pressure. During the course of treatment for the ulcer, he will also need education on the care of his feet and nails, assessment of his understanding of nutrition and glucose control, callus removal from the right foot, and appropriate footwear. After the ulcer is healed on the left foot, he will need appropriate footwear for the left foot as well. As mentioned at the beginning of this chapter, care of the diabetic patient is complex. This is an overview of some of the main concerns of the patient with a diabetic foot ulcer. Prepare before you meet this patient by finding out who your resources are: diabetic specialists, foot clinics, podiatrists, and/or pedorthists.

REFERENCES

Armstrong, D. G., et al. (1998). Risk factors for diabetic foot ulceration: A logical approach to treatment. *Journal of Wound, Ostomy, and Continence Nursing, 25*(3), 123–128.

Elftman, P. (1998). Management of the neuropathic foot. In C. Sussman & B. M. Bates-Jensen (Eds.), *Wound care: A collaborative practice manual for physical therapists and nurses* (pp. 315–345). Gaithersburg, MD: Aspen.

Kelechi, T. J., & Lukas, K. S. (1997). Options in practice: Patient with dystrophic toenails, calluses, and heel fissures. *Journal of Wound, Ostomy, and Continence Nursing, 24*(4), 237–242.

Kelechi, T. J., & Lukas, K. S. (1999). *Basic foot care: A self-instructional manual.* Charleston: Medical University of South Carolina, Center for the Study of Aging.

Kravitz, S. R., McGuire, J., & Shanahan, S. D. (2003). Physical assessment of the diabetic foot. *Advances in Skin & Wound Care, 16*(2), 68–75.

Levin, M. E. (1998). Prevention and treatment of diabetic foot wounds. *Journal of Wound, Ostomy, and Continence Nursing, 25*(3), 129–146.

Levin, M. E., et al. (Eds.). (1993). *The diabetic foot* (5th ed.). St. Louis, MO: Mosby-Year Book.

Mulder, G. A. (2000). Evaluating and managing the diabetes foot: An overview. *Advances in Skin and Wound Care, 13*(1), 33–39.

Steed, D. L. (1997). Diabetic wounds: Assessment, classification and management. In D. Krasner & D. Kane (Eds.), *Chronic wound care: A clinical source book for healthcare professionals* (pp. 172–177). Wayne, PA: Health Management Publications.

BIBLIOGRAPHY

Beuscher, T. L. (2007). Foot and nail care. In R. A. Bryant & D. P. Nix (Eds.), *Acute and chronic wounds: Current management concepts* (3rd ed., pp. 337–360). St. Louis, MO. Mosby Elsevier.

Driver, V. R., et al. (2007). Neuropathic wounds: The diabetic wound. In R. A. Bryant & D. P. Nix (Eds.), *Acute and chronic wounds: Current management concepts* (3d ed., pp. 307–336). St. Louis, MO. Mosby Elsevier.

Frykberg, R. G. (1998). The team approach in diabetic foot management. *Advances in Wound Care, 11*(2), 71–77.

Levin, M. E. (1997). Diabetic foot wounds: Pathogenesis and management. *Advances in Wound Care, 10*(2), 24–30.

Synder, R. S., Cohen, M. M., Sevin, C., & Livingston, J. (2001). Osteomyelitis in the diabetic patient: Diagnosis and treatment part I: Overview, diagnosis and microbiology. *Ostomy Wound Management, 47*(1), 18–30.

RESOURCES

National Diabetes Education Program: Feet Can Last a Lifetime; http://www.ndep.nih.gov

American Diabetes Association, 1701 North Beauregard St., Alexandria, VA 22311; http://www.diabetes.org

American Association of Diabetic Educators, 200 W. Madison St., Suite 800, Chicago, IL 60606; http://www.diabeteseducator.org/

Lavery, L. A., Baranoski, S., & Ayello, E. A. (2000). Diabetic foot ulcers. In S. Baranoski & E. A. Ayello (Eds.), *Wound care essentials: Practice principles* (pp. 311–332). Philadelphia, PA: Lippincott Williams & Wilkins.

Teresa Kelechi, College of Nursing, Medical University of South Carolina, 99 Jonathan Lucas St., Charleston, SC 29425.

Wound, Ostomy and Continence Nurses Society. (2004). *Guidelines for management of wounds in patients with lower-extremity neuropathic disease.* WOCN Clinical Practice Guideline Series No. 3. Glenview, IL. Author.

Skin Tears

Donna Oddo

Skin tears are a common problem in wound care. Minor skin tears can be resolved with minimal intervention. Serious skin tears may lead to large areas of skin loss, fluid imbalances, infections, and sepsis. Long-term complex care, possibly even skin grafts, could be required to achieve closure. They often cause disfigurement and altered body image concerns. Although skin tears may occur anywhere on the body, they are most commonly seen on the upper extremities. It is important to correctly identify and document skin tears and not place them in the category of a pressure ulcer (**Figures 11–1** and **11–2**; **Color Plates 8** and **23**).

Skin tears are most likely to occur on fragile, aged, dry skin. They can be caused by trauma, such as a bump or fall, or by removal of adhesives on the skin. When treating skin tears, caution must be taken to avoid further skin damage by minimizing the use of adhesives.

ETIOLOGY

In normal tissue, dermal and epidermal tissue are firmly meshed. In aging skin, there is:

- decreased collagen
- decreased elasticity
- decreased epidermis thickness
- decreased turgor
- decreased subcutaneous fat

ASSESSMENT

There are four types of tears:

1. flaps
   - viable—integrity restored
   - nonviable—tissue loss results
2. linear (epidermal tissue that can be approximated without loss of coverage)

Figure 11–1 Skin Tear on Lower Extremity. Note fragile "onion peel" type skin surrounding the wound.

Clinical Objectives:

(1) Clean

(2) Protect wound and surrounding tissue

(3) Keep moist

See Color Plate 8.

3. partial-thickness tissue loss (tissue loss involving the epidermis and into but not through the dermis)

4. full-thickness tissue loss (unusual; extends through the epidermis and dermis and into the subcutaneous tissue)

PREVENTION

Patients at Risk

- elderly
- frail
- previous skin tears
- poor nutritional status
- poor hydration status
- poor mobility
- dementia
- history of falls
- history of bruising

Figure 11–2 Skin Tear with 75% of Epidermal Flap Missing.

Clinical Objectives:

(1) Approximate the skin tear flap/tissue as
   closely as possible

(2) Protect wound and surrounding tissue

(3) Keep moist

(4) No tape on skin—nonadherent dressings should be secured with a gauze
   or tubular nonadhesive wrap

See Color Plate 23.

Interventions

See **Exhibit 11–1**.

Intrinsic

- Improve nutritional status.
- Improve hydration status.

Extrinsic

- environment
  - Assess living area for potential hazards.
  - Pad side rails or wheelchair sides.

Exhibit 11–1 How to Stop Skin Tears

Soften the skin; use moisturizers liberally.

Treat new tears promptly.

Optimize the host—a healthy patient is less likely to experience tears.

Protect the arms with sleeves or stockinette.

Safety-check environment for sharp edges, fall hazards.

Keep needed items in reach of patient.

Instruct patient and caregivers in home safety and skin care.

No aggressive adhesives on fragile skin!

Transfer with caution; protect fragile skin from friction.

Encourage fluids.

Assess need for multidisciplinary interventions.

Reevaluate frequently.

Skin tears are preventable!

- mobility
  - Consult physical therapy.
  - Consult occupational therapy.
- protection
  - Moisturize skin.
  - Use sleeves or stockinette.

Education

See **Exhibit 11–2**.

- nutrition and hydration
- safety issues
- protection

TREATMENT CHOICES

Goals

- Prevent further tears.
- Maintain an environment to promote wound healing.
- Prevent trauma to the skin tear by minimizing dressing changes.

Exhibit 11–2 Patient Guide: Preventing and Treating Skin Tears

Aging, certain illnesses, and medications may cause the skin to become dry and fragile. When this happens, any bump or minor injury may cause the skin to open or tear. These skin tears may bleed, become infected, or lead to more serious skin problems. If this is a new problem, seek medical advice to determine the cause of the skin changes.

The following measures may reduce the risk of getting skin tears:

- Eat a well-balanced diet.
- Drink plenty of fluids, especially water.
- Keep skin soft and supple by using only mild soap and by applying a moisturizing cream daily.
- If experiencing balance problems or falls, seek medical advice regarding the cause and about the use of medical equipment to keep you safe (such as walkers or canes).
- Check the home for any sharp hazards. Keep pathways clear.
- Use extra caution in the bathroom. Consider installing grab bars where needed.
- Consider wearing long sleeves to protect your arms.

If you do experience a skin tear, the following measures may be taken:

- Cleanse the wound with mild soap and water. Rinse well with plain water. Pat dry gently with gauze or a clean washcloth.
- Stop the bleeding by applying gentle pressure with gauze or a clean washcloth.
- Apply an antibiotic ointment sparingly to the open wound bed.
- Cover with a nonstick gauze pad.
- Change the dressing each day, cleaning each time with mild soap and water.
- If the wound involves a large area of skin, if the bleeding does not stop quickly, or if signs of infection develop, seek medical advice. Signs of infection include redness and warmth surrounding the wound, change in the color of the drainage, foul odor, fever, or increased discomfort at the site.

Flaps (Viable) or Linear Tears

- Steri-strips—Use caution if more than 24 hours have passed from time of injury or if the injury involved contamination of tissue with "dirty" object.
- Nonadherent dressings.

Partial Thickness Skin Tears

- Antibiotic ointment and nonadherent dressing used together (See Figure 11–2 for step by step instructions.)

- Foam dressing—useful when decreasing frequency of dressing changes, minimizes trauma to surrounding tissue
- Nonadherent dressings, such as hydrogel impregnated gauze/sheet
- Absorbent Tegaderm

Full-Thickness Skin Tears

- Hydrogel impregnated gauze
- Alginates
- Foams
- Surgical intervention (grafting)

CASE STUDY

Mrs. Peters is an 86-year-old white female referred to home health for assessment and management of skin tears on her bilateral upper extremities. They were sustained after a fall in her bathroom.

Examination revealed a frail, thin woman with poor turgor and very dry skin. She was unkempt, stating "my daughter has been taking care of me, but she died last month. I'm not doing too well on my own." Mrs. Peters has a history of mild congestive heart failure for which she took digoxin and furosemide daily.

Dressings (gauze wrap) covered both arms and were held fast to her skin with dried sanguineous drainage. To ease removal and lessen trauma to the skin, the dressings were soaked in saline. On the right forearm, a linear tear was noted, measuring 3 cm long × 4 cm wide × 0 cm deep. The surrounding skin was intact but with a fragile "onion skin" appearance. The left forearm revealed a partial thickness tear 4 cm long × 3 cm wide × 2 cm deep. Neither wound was actively bleeding nor was there any erythema, warmth, or induration. Both sites were cleansed with normal saline, and the intact skin was treated with a protective skin barrier wipe. A transparent film dressing was placed over the linear tear on the right arm. A nonadherent foam dressing was placed over the wound on the left arm and secured in place with gauze wrap. Tubed gauze was applied to both arms for protection from the wrist to above the elbow. A plan of care was established for Mrs. Peters using an interdisciplinary approach. The nurse continued to visit, changing the transparent film dressing weekly and changing the foam dressing three times weekly. The nurse also drew blood for analysis.

Mrs. Peters was then instructed, per physician order, to lower her dose of digoxin and add a potassium supplement. She was taught signs and symptoms of electrolyte imbalance and digoxin toxicity. Her diet teaching stressed the importance of adequate protein, calories, and potassium-rich foods. A home health aide visited three times weekly to assist with personal care and to moisturize Mrs. Peters's dry skin. A physical therapist developed an exercise regimen to help strengthen the patient and enhance her mobility. A walker and a raised toilet seat were obtained; the towel bar (where the left arm injury occurred) was removed as were skid rugs in the bathroom. A social worker assisted with community resources and arranged for private assistance after discharge from home health.

Mrs. Peters was discharged from home health following 6 weeks of care. Both skin tears had healed, and no new tears occurred. She was more mobile, safer, and more secure in her own abilities. A support system had been established within the community.

BIBLIOGRAPHY

Baranoski, S. (2000). Skin tears: The enemy of frail skin. *Advances in Skin & Wound Care, 13*(3), 123–126.

Krasner, D., & Kane, D. (Eds.). (1997). *Chronic wound care: A clinical source book for healthcare professionals* (2d ed.). Wayne, PA: Health Management Publications.

McGough-Csarny, J. (1998). Skin tears in institutionalized elderly: An epidemiological study. *Ostomy/Wound Management, 44*(3A), 145–255.

McTigue, T., et al. (2009). Efficacy of a skin tear education program. *Journal of Wound, Ostomy, and Continence Nursing, 36*(5), 486–492.

Pieper, B., et al. (1999). Wound prevalence, types and treatments in home care. *Advanced Wound Care, 12*(3), 117–125.

Ratliff, C., & Fletcher, K. (2007). Skin tears: A review of the evidence to support prevention and treatment. *Ostomy/Wound Management, 53*, 32–34.

Roberts, M. (2007). Preventing and managing skin tears: A review. *Ostomy/Wound Management, 34*(35), 256–259.

Surgical Wounds and Radiation Burns

Pamela Brown

SURGICAL WOUNDS

Surgical wounds and lacerations are usually closed by primary intention. The wound margins (edges) are brought together soon after the wounding and secured with sutures, staples, or adhesive strips. Wounds closed by primary intention usually heal in 7 to 14 days with minimal scarring (**Figure 12–1**; **Color Plate 24**). Occasionally, such a wound fails to heal properly, resulting in separation of the wound margins and dehiscence or evisceration (**Figures 12–2** and **12–3**; **Color Plates 25** and **26**). These wounds are usually left open to heal by secondary intention. The wound edges contract and decrease the size of the wound while the wound bed fills in with granulation (scar) tissue. Finally epithelialization of the wound surface occurs. This process may take weeks or months. (**Table 12–1**, **Table 12–2** and **Exhibit 12–1**.)

Cleaning the Wound

The surgical wound must be cleansed with each dressing change. Use normal saline with an angiocath and syringe to thoroughly irrigate the wound. A spray saline that can provide a therapeutic pressure or a nonionic surfactant wound cleanser can also be used.

Treatment Choices

Frequency of dressing change depends on the amount and type of wound drainage. The manufacturer's recommendations for products used should be followed.

Exudating Wounds

(These wounds may or may not need debridement.)

- calcium alginate
- hydrofibers
- gauze moistened with normal saline

Figure 12–1 Clean, Granular Surgical Wound with Small Amount of Slough in Center. Note colostomy.
Clinical Objectives:

(1) Clean   (3) Manage exudate
(2) Keep moist   (4) Protect from colostomy drainage
See Color Plate 24.

Figure 12–2 Open Surgical Incision with Tunneling.
Clinical Objectives:

(1) Clean   (3) Manage exudate
(2) Keep moist   (4) Pack tunneling loosely
See Color Plate 25.

Figure 12–3 Necrotic Tissue (Eschar) at Above-Knee Amputation Site of Stump Incision Line. Note erythema and poorly approximated incision line.

Clinical Objectives:

(1) Remove eschar

(2) Clean

(3) Keep moist

(4) Manage exudate

(5) Culture (if appropriate)

See Color Plate 26.

Nonexudating Wounds

Use a dressing that will keep the wound bed moist and clean of necrotic tissue.

- gauze moistened with normal saline
- wound gel or gauze impregnated with gel

> **TIP** Older individuals are at higher risk for poorer healing outcomes. Due to physiologic changes with age, there is decreased elastin in the skin and differences in collagen replacement. The decreased rate of replacement cells affects the rate of wound healing and reepithelialization of the skin

RADIATION BURNS

Radiation triggers changes in the skin that can create ulceration during therapy, immediately after therapy, or years after completion of radiation therapy. Radiation burns initially are shallow, and they may occur spontaneously or in response to trauma. The ulcer is often painful and progressively enlarges to the margins of the irradiated skin field despite optimum treatment.

Table 12–1 Healing Signs for Surgical Wound Healing

Outcome Measure	Days 1 to 4: New Wound	Days 5 to 9: Healing	Days 10 to 14: Proliferative Healing	Day 15 to Years 1–2: New Skin Forming
Incision color	Red, edges approximated	Red, progressing to bright pink (all skin tones)	Bright pink (all skin tones)	Pale pink, progressing to white or silver in light-skinned patients; pale pink, progressing to darker than normal skin color or may blanch to white in dark-skinned patients.
Surrounding tissue inflammation	Swelling, redness, or skin discoloration; warmth, pain	None present	None present	None present
Drainage type	Bloody, progressing to yellow/ clear	None present	None present	None present
Drainage amount	Moderate to minimal	None present	None present	None present
Closure materials	Present, may be sutures or staples	Beginning to remove external sutures/ staples	Sutures/staples removed, Steri-strips or tape strips may be present	None present
New skin	Present by day 4 along entire incision	Present along entire incision	Present	Present
Healing ridge	None present	Present by day 9 along entire incision	Present along entire incision	Present

Source: Reprinted from Bates-Jensen, B. M., & Wethe, J. (1998). Acute Surgical Management. In C. Sussman & B. M. Bates-Jensen (Eds.), *Wound care: A collaborative practice manual for physical therapists and nurses,* (2nd ed. p. 232), Aspen Publishers, Inc.

Treatment

Goals of treatment can be pain control, management of exudate, and odor control (**Exhibit 12–2**).

- Cleanse the wound gently with normal saline.
- Do wound care with wound gel in the form of a sheet (change daily) or amorphous hydrogel (apply three times a day) covered with a nonadherent dressing.

Table 12–2 Unwanted Results for Surgical Wound Healing

Outcome Measure	Days 1 to 4: New Wound	Days 5 to 9: Healing	Days 10 to 14: Proliferative Healing	Day 15 to Years 1–2: New Skin Forming
Incision	Red, edges approximated but tension evident on incision line	Red, edges may not be well approximated; tension on incision line evident	May remain red, progressing to bright pink	Prolonged new skin formation, keloid or hypertrophic scar formation
Surrounding tissue inflammation	No signs of inflammation present: no swelling, no redness or skin discoloration, no warmth, and minimal pain at incision site; hematoma (bruise) formation	Swelling, redness, or skin discoloration; warmth, pain at incision site; hematoma (bruise) formation	Prolonged inflammatory response with swelling, redness, or skin discoloration; warmth and pain; hematoma (bruising) formation	If healing, may be stalled at a plateau with no evidence of healing and continued signs of redness, pus, heat or coolness, pain or numbness
Drainage type	Bloody, progressing to yellow/clear	Red tinged/yellow and pus	Any type of drainage (pus) present	Any type of drainage (pus) present
Drainage amount	Moderate to minimal	Moderate to minimal	Any amount present	Any amount present
Closure materials	Present, may be sutures or staples	No removal of any external sutures/staples	Sutures/staples still present	For secondary intention healing, failure of wound contraction or edges not approximated
New skin	Not present along entire incision	Not present along entire incision	Not present along entire incision, opening of incision line	Not present or abnormal skin appearance, such as keloid or hypertrophic scarring
Healing ridge	None present	Not present along entire incision	Not present along entire incision, opening of incision line	Abscess formation with wound left open to heal slowly

Source: Reprinted from Bates-Jensen, B. M., & Wethe, J. (1998). Acute Surgical Management. In C. Sussman & B. M. Bates-Jensen (Eds.) *Wound care: A collaborative practice manual for physical therapists and nurses,* (2nd ed. p. 230), Aspen.

Exhibit 12–1 Self-Care Guidelines for Acute Surgical Wound Healing

Instructions Given (Date/Initials)	Demonstration or Review of Material (Date/Initials)	Return Demonstration or States Understanding (Date/Initials)

1. Type of incisional wound and specific cautions required
   a. No heavy lifting and other measures to prevent hernia formation
   b. Showering or bathing area
   c. Importance of adequate nutrition for wound healing
2. Significance of wound drainage, incision wound tissue color, surrounding tissue condition, and presence of healing ridge
3. Wound dressing care routine:
   a. Wash hands, then remove old dressing and discard
   b. Clean wound with normal saline
   c. Apply primary dressing to wound
   d. Apply secondary dressing if appropriate
   e. Secure dressing with tape
   f. Practice universal precautions and proper dressing disposal
   g. Follow prescribed frequency of dressing changes
4. Expected change in wound appearance during healing process
   a. Scheduled removal of closure materials
   b. Incision color change as wound heals (bright red or pink to pale pink and finally to silvery white or gray)
5. When to notify the health care provider
   a. Signs and symptoms of wound infection (erythema, edema, pain, elevated temperature, change in drainage character or amount, discoloration in tissues surrounding incision wound)
   b. Absent or incomplete healing ridge along incision after postoperative day 9 at opening of wound incision
6. Importance of follow-up with health care provider		

Note: Must be individualized for each patient and caregiver.
Source: Reprinted from Bates-Jensen, B. M., & Wethe, J. (1998). Acute Surgical Management. In C. Sussman & B. M. Bates-Jenses, (Eds.), *Wound care: A collaborative practice manual for physical therapists and nurses,* (2nd ed. p. 229), Aspen.

- Do not use tape on the skin. Use soft net, soft stretch net briefs, or tailor cotton jersey underpants or undershirts to hold the dressing in place. Do not use dressings that adhere to the wound or to the surrounding radiation-damaged skin.

TIP If the patient is still undergoing radiation treatment, it is important to use products that will not interfere with radiation therapy. Most wound products cannot be used while the patient is undergoing radiation therapy. Do not use any product on the radiated skin until you have checked with the physician.

Exhibit 12–2 Patient Guide: What Happens to the Skin During Radiation Therapy Treatment?

While you are receiving radiation therapy, one of the areas you and your radiation oncology team will be monitoring is your skin and the effects the radiation is having on it.

- The specific area of the body to be treated is called the treatment field.
- The cancer cells within the field are treated with radiation therapy that is administered through the skin. The skin needs special care during the treatment period.
- Radiation therapy makes the skin in the treatment field very dry. Therefore, it becomes very susceptible to skin irritations.
- The severity of skin reactions varies from person to person. One or more of the following changes can occur in the treatment field:
  - slowly increasing redness
  - dry, peeling skin
  - itching
  - swelling
  - hot sensation
  - rashes
  - blistering
  - moist, weepy areas
  - decreased perspiration
  - hair loss
  - thinning of skin

YOUR SKIN CARE IN THE TREATMENT FIELD DURING AND AFTER RADIATION THERAPY

Important: Do not remove markings on skin until instructed to do so.

Cleansing

1. Cleanse hair and body per normal routine or as recommended using mild, gentle products.

(continues)

Exhibit 12–2 *continued*

2. Use a soft washcloth to gently cleanse the treatment field—DO NOT RUB THE SKIN.
3. Rinse area and PAT dry
   Recommended shampoo, cleanser/soap: _____

Moisturizing

1. Gently apply lotion or cream to treatment field.
2. Repeat moisturizing two to three times daily.
3. Use only prescribed creams or lotions in treatment field.
4. Begin moisturizing after first treatment and continue as recommended. Recommended moisturizers:

Long-Term Care of Skin in Treatment Field

• Moisturize area every day with a recommended cream or lotion.
• Protect from the sun using a sunblock with an SPF 15 or higher.
• Protect from irritations that can be caused by:
  • *chemicals* such as cleaning solutions or solvents
  • *mechanical irritation* such as continuous rubbing of belts or tight clothing
  • *physical irritation* such as extreme heat and cold, or cuts and scrapes

Source: Courtesy of Coloplast Corporation, 2000, Marietta, GA.

BIBLIOGRAPHY

Cooper, D. (1992). Acute surgical wounds. In R. Bryant (Ed.), *Acute and chronic wounds* (pp. 91–100). St. Louis, MO: Mosby-Year Book.

Kane, D. (1997). Surgical repair. In D. Krasner & D. Kane (Eds.), *Chronic wound care: A clinical source book for health care professionals* (2d ed., pp. 235–244). Wayne, PA: Health Management Publications.

Mendelsohn, F. A., et al. (2002). Wound care after radiation therapy. *Advances in Skin & Wound Care, 15*(5), 216–224.

Mulder, D., et al. (1998). *Clinician's pocket guide to chronic wound repair.* Springhouse, PA: Springhouse Corporation.

Porock, D., et al. (1999). Management of radiation skin reactions: Literature review and clinical application. *Plastic Surgical Nursing, 19*(4), 185–192.

Supple, K. G. (2004). Physiologic response to burn injury. In *Critical Care Nurse Clinician, 16*(1):119.

Wysocki, A., & Bryant R. (1992). Skin. In R. Bryant (Ed.), *Acute and chronic wounds: Nursing management* (pp. 1–25). St. Louis, MO: Mosby-Year Book.

Palliative Wound Care Approaches

MariJo Letizia

Patients may experience wounds at or near the end of life that are difficult to treat and may not be amenable to healing. In these cases, hospice and palliative care may be considered. Palliative care approaches include stabilization of existing wounds, prevention of new wounds, and symptom management with a focus on quality of life. Treatment goals for nonhealing wounds at the end of life include managing wound exudate, controlling odor, maximizing mobility and function, preventing wound infection, and controlling pain and other symptoms. In addition to wound care strategies, other components of palliative care include communication and psychosocial support for patients and families.

INTRODUCTION

Providers who care for seriously ill patients with life-threatening illness recognize the many challenges with this population. One aspect of care that can be particularly difficult is the management of nonhealing wounds. Chronic, nonhealing wounds are defined as any interruption in the continuity of the skin that either requires longer than a 6-month period of time to heal, or fail to heal (Kranke, Bennett, Roeckl-Wiedmann, & Debus, 2006). Such wounds are common as patients approach the end of life; for example, up to 28% of those in long-term care and hospice programs will experience a pressure ulcer (Alvarez, et al., 2007). These patients also may experience arterial ulcers, malignant wounds, and venous ulcerations.

Patients who have transitioned to palliative care may experience wounds that are directly related to an advanced disease state (Naylor, 2005). In this patient population, the skin is both vulnerable to breakdown and less able to heal (Langemo, 2005). A number of factors are involved in such skin changes, including diminished mobility and reduced intake of fluid and food as patients decline. Perfusion of oxygen and delivery of nutrients to the tissues can be diminished, and protein synthesis can be impaired in the presence of increased catabolic processes (Langemo). With these factors, complete wound healing and wound closure may

Letizia, M., Uebelhor, J., & Paddack, E. (2010). Providing palliative care to seriously ill patients with non-healing wounds. *Journal of Wound, Ostomy, and Continence Nursing, 37*(3), 277–284.

not be possible. Also, as the dying process progresses, patients with increasingly frail skin may develop Kennedy Terminal Ulcers on various pressure points. These ulcers can occur suddenly and are associated with rapid skin deterioration, at times resulting in stage III-IV wounds (Schim & Cullen, 2005).

In managing wounds of patients receiving palliative care approaches, aggressive interventions that are focused on cure may no longer be appropriate or desired by patients and their families. Instead, priorities shift to stabilizing the wound, preventing new wounds, and managing symptoms with a focus on the quality of the patient's life.

PALLIATIVE CARE: GENERAL PRINCIPLES

According to the World Health Organization (WHO), palliative care is defined as the active, total care of patients whose disease is not responsive to curative treatment (Fleck, 2005). The palliative care philosophy regards dying as a normal process. Interventions are directed at preventing, reducing, and relieving symptoms of disease or disorders, rather than curative treatment approaches. Both the patient and family are considered the unit of care. Within this philosophical framework, care is provided by interdisciplinary team members up through the time of bereavement.

In the United States, hospice is a component of palliative care. Hospice and palliative care are both appropriate when there is little likelihood of cure for the patient's underlying disease. Although seriously ill patients living with incurable illnesses can and should receive care focused on palliation, only those patients with a 6-month life expectancy can qualify for hospice services (Schim & Cullen, 2005). Reimbursement mechanisms for hospice care include the Hospice Medicare Benefit (MHB), state Medicaid benefit, and private insurance/HMO benefits.

INDICATIONS FOR PALLIATIVE WOUND CARE APPROACHES

One trigger for identification of patients who might benefit from palliative wound care approaches has been suggested by William Ennis, who encourages providers to ask the following question: "Would this patient's life be significantly better, from a quality-of-life standpoint, if the wound was healed?" (Ennis & Meneses, 2005). Ennis believes that if the answer to this question is "no," then palliative care should be considered. Reasonable palliative care goals, all related to the quality of life, include reducing the number of hospitalizations while maintaining comfort at home; forgoing life-sustaining treatment; and discontinuing elements of the plan of care that do not contribute to comfort. Although palliative care includes attention to psychosocial and spiritual concerns and physical needs of the patient, it also incorporates the family and family concerns in the plan of care. Specifically regarding wounds that are present at the end of life, attention is directed to the feelings of embarrassment, depression, anxiety, and social isolation that may be experienced (McDonald & Lesage, 2006).

The FRAIL (For Recognition of the Adult Immobilized Life) program provides another mechanism to help providers identify patients who have wounds that are unlikely to heal and who, along with family members, will benefit from palliative care (Tice, 2006).[9] This model emphasizes the wishes and priorities of the patient, so that strategies for wound management are adjusted to those stated goals. Of note, the FRAIL model urges providers to accept nonhealing endpoints as appropriate and in the best interest of many frail patients.

Criteria established in the FRAIL model focus holistically on the patient's physical, psychological, social, and spiritual variables (Fleck, 2005). The FRAIL model's Healing Probability Assessment Tool includes data related to the patient's wounds as well as nutrition and activity level (**Table 13–1**). Variables identified in this tool are similar to the criteria for hospice using the diagnosis "Debility, unspecified" (**Table 13–2**). Both the Healing Probability Assessment Tool and the established criteria for the hospice diagnosis of "Debility, unspecified" contain objective parameters indicative of deteriorating health indicating that the individual may benefit from palliative care.

PALLIATIVE CARE: COMMUNICATION ISSUES

When identifying patients who may be appropriate for palliative care, it is essential to consider communication approaches with the patient and family. Because many people may make the assumption that all wounds are able to fully heal, a

Table 13–1 Healing Probability Assessment Tool

- Wound is over 3 months old or is a recurrence of a preexisting breakdown
- Patient spends 20 or more hours per day in a dependent position
- Patient is incontinent of urine
- Patient has loss greater than 5% of baseline weight, or 10 pounds, in the past 90 days
- Patient does not eat independently
- Patient does not walk independently
- Patient has a history of falls within the last 90 days
- Patient is unable/unwilling to avoid placing weight over wound(s) site(s)
- Wound is associated with complications of diabetes mellitus
- Wound is associated with peripheral vascular disease
- Severe chronic obstructive pulmonary disease
- End stage renal, liver, or heart disease
- Wound is associated with arterial disease
- Patient has diminished range of motion (ROM) status nonresponsive to rehabilitative services
- Patient has diminished level of mental alertness demonstrated by muted communication skills and inability to perform activities of daily living (ADLs) independently
- Wound is full thickness with presence of tunneling
- Blood values indicate low oxygen carrying capacity
- Blood values indicate an exhausted or decreased immune capacity
- Blood values indicate below normal visceral protein levels that have not responded to nutritional support efforts

Table 13–2 Criteria for Determining Terminal Status as Stated under the Medical Guidelines for Determining Prognosis: Decline in Health (ICD9 code 799.3)

- Progression of disease as documented by symptoms, signs, and test results provided below
- Decline in Karnofsky Perfomance Score and Palliative Performance Score
- Evidence of unintentional, progressive weight loss of >10% over the prior 6 months:
  - Provide weight and/or muscle mass history as above
  - If available, document these additional markers of nutritional status include:
    - Serum albumin less than 2.5 gm/dl or
    - Combination of serum cholesterol under 156 mg/dl and Hct less than 41 mg/dl
- Dependence on assistance for two or more activities of daily living
- Dysphagia leading to inadequate nutritional intake as evidenced by findings documented below
- Decline in systolic BP relative to the patient's baseline reading or progressive postural hypotension
- Evidence of the increasing need for skilled service
- Decline in Functional Assessment Staging (FAST) for dementia
- Progressive stage 3-4 pressure ulcers in spite of optimal care

discussion with the patient and family may initially focus on the likely possibility that the wound is unlikely to heal. Emphasis can be placed on the fact that such a nonhealing wound is a symptom of declining health, and that this situation is likely not a reflection of failure on the part of the patient, family, or provider. These discussions help reduce a caregiver's feeling of blame or incompetence (Advanced Medical Technology Association, 2006). With a focus on realistic outcomes in light of advanced disease, reasonable treatment options can be outlined. It is important to validate that the patient and family have understood information that is given regarding assessment of the situation and treatment options. The provider should also ensure that they have heard and understood the perspectives of the patient and family in terms of goals of care and decisions about treatment.

The words "hospice" and "palliative care" may evoke feelings of concern in patients and family members. Some may consider these approaches as "throwing in the towel" or "giving up hope"; and others may believe that by suggesting hospice and palliative care, the provider may be abandoning the patient (Alvarez, et al., 2007). In fact, end-of-life care is not synonymous with end of care; instead, the focus shifts away from aggressive interventions intended to cure to aggressive interventions intended to provide comfort. Therefore, providers are encouraged to avoid inaccurate statements such as "there is nothing more we can do for you."

WOUND MANAGEMENT IN PALLIATIVE CARE

The transition to palliative care for patients with nonhealing wounds involves a clear focus on strategies to stabilize the wound(s) and prevent the development of new wounds; complete wound healing may not be a feasible goal. With that in mind, a number of general considerations form the basis for specific interventions, including managing exudate, controlling odor, maximizing mobility and function, preventing infection, and controlling pain and other symptoms (Lee, Ennis, & Dunn, 2007). The rationale for maintaining moist wound healing properties in traditional wound care is well established (Brett, 2006). These principles are also maintained in the palliative care setting, because it helps to stabilize the wound and reduce tissue trauma and pain during dressing changes.

Managing Wound Exudate

The wound and periwound skin are thoroughly assessed to determine topical therapy needs based on the characteristics of the wound(s). Key assessment includes the wound depth, presence of tunneling or undermining, volume of exudate, and the need for a bacterial barrier. The volume of wound exudates is a key assessment that has a profound impact on the selection of an appropriate category of dressing (see **Table 13–3**). Over 200 product manufacturers market various brands of wound products and dressings related to wound exudate management. Protection of the periwound skin from damage due to exposure to exudates is an additional goal of care. Prevention of periwound maceration includes selection of wound dressings that absorb exudates and minimize trauma to the adjacent skin during dressing changes. For further protection, an ointment-based or polymer acrylate skin protectant may be applied with each dressing change or as indicated.

Managing Wound Odor

Wound odor can be a source of great distress for the patient and his/her family, resulting in feelings of embarrassment, disgust, depression, and leading to social isolation (McManus, 2007). General approaches to combat wound odor include the following: using a room deodorizer, promptly disposing of old wound dressings, and performing frequent dressing changes. External odor absorbers (such as kitty litter or vinegar) placed at or near the bed may also aid in the elimination of odor, wherever the patient is residing. Although charcoal-activated dressings are expensive, reduction in wound odor can also be achieved by applying them directly to the wound. The following factors are associated with increased wound odor: bacterial burden or infection in the wound, the presence of necrotic material, the presence of fungating malignant tumors, and poor wound care practices(McDonald & Lesage, 2006; Paul & Pieper, 2008).

Colonization or infection with the following organisms contributes to wound odor: *Bacteroides fragilis*, *Bacteroides prevotella*, *Fusobacterium nucleatum*, *Clostridium perfringens*, *Proteus spp.*, *Pseudomonas spp.*, and *Klebsiella spp* (Alvarez, et al., 2007). To combat infection and the resulting odor, products with impregnated silver are useful; these can be selectively toxic to microorganisms such as bacteria

Table 13–3 Managing Wound Exudate in the Palliative Care Setting

Exudate	Dressing	Types	Advantages in Palliative Care Setting
Light to Moderate	Hydrogel	Water or glycerin based amorphous gels, impregnated gauzes or sheet dressings.	Increase epidermal healing, enhance autolytic debridement of slough, and soothes while reduces pain (Alvarez, et al., 2007).
	Hydrocolloid	Gelatin, pectin, and carboxy-methylcellulose that are manufactured in various shapes, sizes, and adhesive properties.	Reduces airborne distribution of organisms at dressing change, self- adherent, and molds well to the body (Brett, 2006).
	Composite/ Clear Acrylic	Patented, clear, acrylic polymer pads with breathable, water-proof clear film layer that are manufactured in various shapes and sizes.	Exudate is contained within the two chambers of the dressing through the process of diffu-sion, decreasing periwound maceration. Clear layer allows for visualization of wound without removal of dressing (Lee, Ennis, & Dunn, 2007).
Moderate to Heavy	Alginate	Calcium salts of alginic acid derived from brown seaweed that forms a gel upon contact with wound fluid. Manufactured in rope or sheet dressings.	Capacity to absorb up to 20 times its weight, which reduces the need for frequent dressing changes (Lee, Ennis, & Dunn, 2007).
	Hydrofiber	Carboxmethylcellulose fibers that form a gel upon contact with wound fluid. Manufactured in rope or sheet dressings.	Capacity to absorb up to 33% more than alginate dressings, which reduces the need for frequent dressing changes (Lee, Ennis, & Dunn, 2007).
	Foam	Vary in thickness. Manufactured as pads, sheets, and pillow cavity dressings. Some types contain additives such as sur-factant and/or glycerin.	May be utilized as a secondary dressing for heavily exudative wounds or under compression wrap therapy (Lee, Ennis, & Dunn, 2007).
Heavy	Negative Pressure Wound Therapy (NPWT)		No reimbursement in the palliative care setting. May use if individual or family is willing to pay out of pocket.

including methicillin-resistant *Staphylococcus aureus* (MRSA), gentamicin-resistant *Pseudomonas spp.*, and *Enterococcus spp.*, as well as various fungal species (White, Cutting, & Kingsley, 2006). Mupirocin ointment is useful in *Staphylococcus aureus* and *Strep pyrogenes* infections. Triple antibiotic ointments may inhibit coagulase-negative *Staphylococci*, *P. aeruginosa*, and *Enterobacteriaceae* infection (White, Cutting, & Kingsley). Malodorous wounds colonized or infected with *Pseudomonas aeruginosa* can be treated with Dakin's (hypochlorite) solution, which has been found to neutralize odors. This treatment is administered locally at ¼ strength twice daily for up to 5 days, and should be discontinued when the odor is eliminated (Alvarez, et al., 2007). Dressings that contain active leptospermum honey also can decrease bacterial burden and odor, both of which are appropriate goals in the palliative care setting; these dressings may also reduce inflammation and aid in autolysis of necrotic tissue (Gunes & Eser, 2007).

Topical and oral metronidazole reduces odor associated with anaerobic infection (McManus, 2007). However, its use for this indication is off label, as efficacy has not been confirmed in randomized, controlled studies. Nevertheless, several studies reported desirable results using topical metronidazole, 0.75% or 0.8%, applied to the wound base then covered with moist saline gauze or dry gauze dressings (McManus). Alternatively, oral metronidazole can be prescribed, dosed at 400 mg three times daily but reduced to 200 mg three times daily or 400 mg daily if the patient experiences nausea (Clinical Knowledge Summaries, 2009). Based on clinical experience, a 250 mg tablet of metronidazole can be crushed and mixed in 2 ounces of 0.9 normal saline, which can then be sprayed directly onto the wound two to three times daily for 5 to 7 days.

Conservative sharp debridement of nonviable tissue may be a reasonable treatment to combat wound odor in the palliative care setting. Application of the enzymatic agent collagenase is an alternative method for debriding a malodorous wound containing necrotic tissue (McCallon & Hurlow, 2009).

Addressing Mobility and Function

In addition to palliative approaches regarding the wound itself, interventions that maximize mobility and function in patients with nonhealing wounds must also be considered, on a case by case basis. Efforts should be initiated to allow the patient to maintain a maximum level of independence for as long as possible. For example, physical and occupational therapy may be indicated for those patients without significant impairment in functional status. It may also be appropriate to lift activity restrictions related to the wound, such as limitations in weight bearing. In all cases, providers must monitor the patient for discomfort or distress during activity and amend the plan to include pain management approaches and/or adjusting the amount and level of activity.

Palliative care patients who are or become bed bound should be provided with pressure redistribution bed support surfaces (Centers for Medicare and Medicaid Services [CMS], 2006). Such support surfaces are grouped into categories, as follows. Group 1 devices provide static pressure reduction; these include foam, gel, and water products, as well as the least expensive air mattresses (McCallon & Hurlow, 2009). In accordance with qualification for reimbursement, the patient must have limited mobility and one accompanying factor related to the wound and healing, such as incontinence. Group 2 devices provide pressure relief by eliminating the external load upon a specific body part. Devices in this group include (1) mattress replacements, (2) mattress overlays, (3) therapy beds that provide static dry flotation, (4) alternating pressure mattresses, (5) kinetic (tilting) therapy, and (6) low air loss mattresses with humidity and temperature controls. Patients who have used group 1 products with development or progression of a wound qualify for the group 2 surfaces. Only one device is listed in Group 3, the Clinitron Air Fluidized Therapy by Hill-Rom, Canton, Massachusetts. This bed is designed for use in the home or institutional setting, to relieve pressure on wound site(s), allowing for increased capillary blood flow while minimizing shear, friction, and maceration (Hill-Rom, 2009). Medicare reimbursement for this support surface is reserved for severely immobile patients who require institutionalization, have stage III or IV pressure ulcer, and/or have failed therapy with any group 2 device. An additional qualifier for home patients is that the patient must have a caregiver who can manage both the patient and the bed (CMS, 2006).

Preventing and Managing Wound Infection

Prevention and management of wound infection is another important consideration in the palliative management of patients with nonhealing wounds. Increased concentrations of bacterial colonies in the wound bed negatively affect wound healing (McManus, 2007; White, Cutting, & Kingsley, 2006). Empiric treatment using topical products with antimicrobial properties, regular wound bed cleansing, and exudates management is indicated when evidence of increased bacterial bioburden is present.

Diagnostic testing, including obtaining a culture/sensitivity in the palliative care patient with a likely wound infection, may be ordered if the results are likely to change the treatment plan, including selection of antibiotic therapy. Of note, osteomylitis is a particularly complex problem in the palliative care population. When wound healing is the primary goal of care, treatment of osteomyelitis usually involves a lengthy course of intravenous antibiotics and possible surgical debridement (Concia, et al., 2006). However, these aggressive interventions that are based on a model of curative care may not provide significant benefit or achieve intended goals in patients receiving palliative care (Lee, Ennis, & Dunn, 2007). Providers must carefully consider both the benefits as well as burdens of treatment when discussing management approaches with patients and their families. In particular, treatments or procedures that are not likely to be effective or benefit the patient should not be imposed (Brock, 2008). Likewise, patients have the autonomous right to refuse treatment, including burdensome or uncomfortable wound care approaches.

Surgical debridement of wounds is undertaken only in selected patients. For example, debridement is avoided in patients with full-thickness heel pressure covered by stable eschar. Nevertheless, surgical debridement may be considered based on the extent of necrotic materials and infection in the wound, the underlying wound pathogenesis, and the patient's likely survival based on perioperative risk factors (European Wound Management Association, 2002).

Controlling Pain

As with all patients receiving hospice and palliative care, pain management is a primary focus for patients who have nonhealing wounds. Wound-associated pain may be associated with a number of factors; it occurs especially during dressing removal (European Wound Management Association, 2002; Woo & Sibbald, 2009). Because of the frequency and severity of pain associated with dressing removal, patients should be premedicated before dressing changes with a quick-acting opioid medication, even if chronic pain is being managed with a long-acting analgesic. Although tolerance to, and dependence on, opioid medications are expected in patients who require them for pain management, concern about addiction is not warranted (Leleszi & Lewandowski, 2005). If patients experience feelings of anxiety with upcoming dressing changes, both pharmacologic and nonpharmacologic approaches to reduce anxiety can also be provided.

Topical anesthestics such as lidocaine EMLA cream are also used to control pain associated with dressing change (McDonald & Lesage, 2006; Woo & Sibbald, 2009). Other strategies to reduce pain related to dressing changes include selecting products that can be removed from the wound with minimal trauma to local tissues and products requiring less frequent dressing changes. Dry dressings should be moistened before removal with a wound cleanser or saline to reduce pain during the dressing removal. Products that provide peri-wound protection can be used to reduce pain from inflammation of surrounding tissue. Tape alternatives are important for those patients with tape sensitivity and particularly fragile tissue, because adhesive tapes and dressings may result in removal of one or more layers of the stratum corneum. Such epidermal stripping occurs with repeated application and removal of adhesive products. Alternatively, nonadherent dressings can be used to maintain a moist wound environment while reducing wound trauma and pain experienced when the dressing is removed. For example, hydrogel dressings may soothe the skin and wounds; cooling effects can be experienced if these dressings are refrigerated prior to application. For moderate to heavily exudative wounds, products that convert to a gel form upon contact with drainage in the wound may be lessen trauma to wound during dressing changes (See Table 13–3).

In addition to pain control, attention must also be paid to managing the multitude of other symptoms that may cause distress to the palliative care patient (McDonald & Lesage, 2006). For example, it is well recognized that dyspnea, nausea, and fatigue often occur at or near the end of life. Ongoing assessment of both pain and nonpain symptoms is crucial in order to implement and then monitor effectiveness of interventions. Patient and family teaching and support are crucial, and care is coordinated with members of the interdisciplinary team.

CONCLUSION

Many palliative care patients experience wounds that are difficult to treat or not amenable to healing. Palliative care approaches in the management of these wounds include stabilizing the wound, preventing new wounds, and managing symptoms with a focus on quality of life. Particular treatment approaches of nonhealing wounds at the end of life include managing wound exudate, controlling odor, maximizing mobility and function, preventing wound infection, and controlling pain and other symptoms. In addition to wound care strategies, other components of palliative care include careful communication with patients and families, as well as psychosocial support.

REFERENCES

Advanced Medical Technology Association. (2006). Advanced wound management: Healing and restoring lives. Retrieved October 18, 2011 from http://www.advamed.org/NR/rdonlyres/8D8348E8-811D-48A9-8737-61D91060DDAD/0/june2006_woundmanagement.pdf

Alvarez, O., Kalinski, C., Nusbaum, J., Hernandez, L., Pappous, E., Kyriannis, C., et al., (2007). Incorporating wound healing strategies to improve palliation (symptom management) in patients with chronic wounds. Journal of Palliative Medicine, 10(5), 1161–1189.

Brett, D. W. (2006). Impact on exudates management, maintenance of a moist wound environment, and prevention of infection. Journal of Wound, Ostomy, and Continence Nursing, 33, 59–64.

Brock, D. (2008). Conscientious refusal by physicians and pharmacists: who is obligated to do what, and why? Theoretical Medicine and Bioethics, 29(3), 187–200.

Centers for Medicare and Medicaid. (2006). Pressure reducing support surfaces. Retrieved September 6, 2008 from http://www.ngsmedicare.com

Clinical Knowledge Summaries. (2009). Palliative cancer care—malignant ulcer of the skin. Retrieved October 18, 2011 from http://www.cks.nhs.uk/palliative_cancer_care_malignant_ulcer

Concia, E., Prandini, N., Massari, L., Ghisellini, F., Consoli, V., Menichetti, F., et al. (2006). Osteomyelitis: clinical update for practical guidelines. Nuclear Medicine Communications, 27, 645–660.

Ennis, W., & Meneses, P. (2005). Palliative care and wound care: Two emerging fields with similar needs for outcomes data. Wounds, 17(4), 99–104.

European Wound Management Association. (2002). Position document: Pain at wound dressing changes. London: Medical Education Partnership.

Fleck, C. (2005). Ethical wound management for the palliative patient. Extended Care Product News, 100(4), 38–46.

FRAIL Palliative Wound Care. (n.d.). Palliative wound care and healing probability assessment tool. Retrieved September 11, 2009 from http://www.frailcare.org /images/Palliative%20Wound%20Care.pdf

Gunes, U. Y., & Eser, I. (2007). Effectiveness of a honey dressing for healing pressure ulcers. *Journal of Wound, Ostomy, and Continence Nursing, 34*, 184–189.

Hill-Rom. (2009). Clinitron air fluidized therapy. Retrieved September 11, 2009 from www.hillrom.com

Kranke, P., Bennett, M., Roeckl-Wiedmann, I., & Debus, S. (2006). Hyperbaric oxygen therapy for chronic wounds [review]. *The Cochrane Collaboration, Database of Systemic Reviews, 1*.

Langemo, D. (2005). When the goal is palliative care. *Advances in Skin & Wound Care, 19*(3), 148–154.

Lee, K., Ennis, W., & Dunn, G. (2007). Surgical palliative care of advanced wounds. *American Journal of Hospice & Palliative Medicine, 24*(2), 154–160.

Leleszi, J., & Lewandowski, J. (2005). Pain management in end-of-life care. *Journal of the American Osteopathic Association, 105*(3), S6–S11.

McCallon, S. K., & Hurlow, J. (2009). Clinical applications for the use of enzymatic debriding ointment and broad spectrum antibacterial foam dressing. *Journal of Wound, Ostomy, and Continence Nursing, 36*(6, Suppl.), S17–S24.

McDonald, A., & Lesage, P. (2006). Palliative management of pressure ulcers and malignant wounds in patients with advanced illness, *Journal of Palliative Medicine, 9*(2), 285–296.

McManus, J. (2007). Principles of skin and wound care: The palliative approach. *End of Life Care, 1*(1), 8–19.

Naylor, W. (2005). A guide to wound management in palliative care. *International Journal of Palliative Nursing, 11*, 572–579.

Paul, J., & Pieper, B. (2008). Topical metronidazole for the treatment of wound odor: a review of the literature. *Ostomy/Wound Management, 54*(3), 18–27.

Schim, S., & Cullen, B. (2005). Wound care at end of life. *Nursing Clinics of North America, 40*(2), 281–294.

Tice, M. (2006). Wound care in the face of life-limiting illness. *Home Health Nurse Care, 24*(2), 115–118.

White, R. J., Cutting, K., & Kingsley, A. (2006). Topical antimicrobials in the control of wound bioburden. *Ostomy Wound Management, 52*(8), 26–58.

Woo, K. Y., & Sibbald, R. G. (2009). The improvement in wound-associated pain and healing trajectory with a comprehensive foot and leg ulcer care model. *Journal of Wound, Ostomy, and Continence Nursing, 36*(2), 184–191.

Specific Applications
of Wound Care Practice

Documentation and Compliance in Home Health Care

Ben Peirce

Documentation requirements for certified home healthcare agencies are largely determined by the Centers for Medicare and Medicaid Services (CMS) conditions of participation and billing requirements. Home health care for patients with commercial insurance is organized differently but generally follows Medicare guidelines. This begins with establishing a realistic plan of care based on a comprehensive assessment done on admission to the home healthcare agency. For patients with wounds, the plan of care must include specific physician's orders for the wound care to be provided on subsequent visits including a complete list of supplies needed. The plan of care must also be updated to reflect all changes in physician's orders and any new supplies needed to follow these orders.

Key components to include in each visit note are assessment of patient condition, description of any treatment or education provided, how the patient responded, status of the home environment, and any communication with the physician and other members of the patient's care team. The description of the treatment should clearly describe the procedure performed and the medical supplies used to substantiate the medical necessity of both the treatment and the supplies. On an ongoing basis, documentation of wound status must clearly show that the patient is making progress toward the goals established in the plan of care and should include wound location, size and depth, drainage type and amount, and condition of wound bed and surrounding skin. Otherwise, coverage for services may be at risk for denial of payment by the payer.

Trends in wound care in the home include:

- focus on objective wound assessment and documentation to demonstrate progress
- screening every patient on admission for risk of pressure ulcer development, obtaining orders, and implementing interventions for those who are at risk
- use of protocols or pathways with time frames to guide establishing goals selecting interventions to support the goals
- use of follow-up case conferences periodically to reevaluate care

Since October 2000, payment for services by CMS is based on the Outcome and Assessment Information Set (OASIS) data that are collected at the start of home health care, transfer, resumption of care, and discharge. Payment is calculated based on OASIS and covers 60 days of service regardless of how many visits or what type of supplies are provided. The amount a home care agency receives from the CMS varies significantly depending on the patient's clinical condition, functional level, and the use of therapy services.

The OASIS data set is generated from the assessment done by the admitting nurse or therapist using a standardized set of questions and must be supported by other assessment information documented in the medical record. Together, these two components form the initial skilled assessment that is the basis of the home health plan of care, also known as the HCFA Form 485. This information must be transmitted electronically to the CMS on admission after hospitalization and discharge in order to be paid for services. Because all reimbursement is based on the OASIS assessment data, clinicians and their managers now understand that accurate assessment is critical to successful home health care. In addition to using OASIS as the basis for payment, CMS also compares patient condition at discharge to condition at admission to identify OASIS-related patient outcomes, reports these to the public and instructs state surveyors to use the data to help guide the survey process. CMS also plans to eventually use OASIS-based outcomes as the basis for payment as part of an initiative known as "pay for performance."

The CMS created the Home Health Compare website of OASIS-based outcomes as a way to provide consumers with an objective basis for selecting a home healthcare agency. For this reason, it is important to answer OASIS questions accurately. Of special note are questions on primary and secondary diagnoses. Not only do these questions on diagnostic coding impact payment, but they are the basis of the plan of care. Their accuracy ensures that the plan of care addresses underlying disease that must be managed to heal wounds and to prevent their recurrence.

When CMS first implemented the prospective payment system in home health care, early feedback from clinicians suggested that the OASIS questions on wound status were difficult to answer because the terminology lacked universal definitions (fully granulating, early/partial granulation, nonhealing). In response to these issues, the Wound, Ostomy and Continence Nurses Society (WOCN) identified and validated definitions in the OASIS guidance document (**Exhibit 14–1**) that was accepted by CMS as appropriate for use when answering OASIS questions. The OASIS guidance document can be a valuable addition to OASIS training tools for home health agencies.

In addition to being skilled at OASIS assessments, clinicians must also be skilled at describing wounds in a narrative note or on wound assessment forms because the OASIS data set alone is not adequate to meet the requirements for a skilled assessment in a certified home health agency.

Exhibit 14–1 Wound, Ostomy and Continence Nurses Society Guidance on Oasis Skin and Wound Status M0 Items

OVERVIEW AND BACKGROUND

As mandated by the Balanced Budget Act of 1997, Home Health Reimbursement shifted to a prospective payment system effective October 2000. Under this system, payment is based on the patient's clinical severity, functional status, and therapy requirements. The system for wound classification uses terms such as "nonhealing," "partially granulating," and "fully granulating"; these terms lack universal definition and clinicians have verbalized concerns that they may be interpreting these terms incorrectly. The WOCN Society has therefore developed the following guidelines for classification of wounds. These items were developed by consensus among the WOCN's panel of content experts.

M0445:	Does the patient have a Pressure Ulcer?
M0450:	Current number of Pressure Ulcers at Each Stage
M0460:	Stage of Most Problematic (Observable) Pressure Ulcer

    1   Stage I
    2   Stage II
    3   Stage III
    4   Stage IV
    NA No observable pressure ulcer

Definitions:

Pressure Ulcer: Any lesion caused by unrelieved pressure resulting in damage of underlying tissue. Shear and friction may be contributing factors. Pressure ulcers are usually located over bony prominences and are staged to classify the degree of tissue damage observed.

- *Stage I:* Non-blanchable erythema of intact skin, the heralding lesion of skin ulceration. In individuals with darker skin, discoloration of the skin, warmth, edema, induration, or hardness may also be indicators.
- *Stage II:* Partial thickness skin loss involving epidermis, dermis, or both. The ulcer is superficial and presents as an abrasion, blister, or shallow crater.
- *Stage III:* Full thickness skin loss involving damage to or necrosis of subcutaneous tissue that may extend down to, but not through, underlying fascia. The ulcer presents clinically as a deep crater with or without undermining of adjacent tissue.
- *Stage IV:* Full thickness skin loss with extensive destruction, tissue necrosis, or damage to muscle, bone, or supporting structures (e.g., tendon, joint capsule). Undermining and sinus tracts (tunnels) may also be associated with Stage IV pressure ulcers.
- *Non-observable:* Wound is unable to be visualized due to an orthopedic device, dressing, etc. A pressure ulcer cannot be accurately staged until the deepest viable tissue layer is visible; *this means that wounds covered with eschar and/or slough cannot be staged, and should be documented as non-observable.*

M0464:	Status of Most Problematic (Observable) Pressure Ulcer

    1   Fully granulating
    2   Early/partial granulation
    3   Not healing
    NA No observable pressure ulcer

(continues)

Exhibit 14–1   *continued*

Definitions:

- *Fully granulating:*
  - wound bed filled with granulation tissue to the level of the surrounding skin or new epithelium
  - no dead space
  - no avascular tissue (eschar and/or slough)
  - no signs or symptoms of infection
  - wound edges are open
- *Early/partial granulation:*
  - ≥25% of the wound bed is covered with granulation tissue
  - there is minimal avascular tissue (eschar and/or slough) (i.e., < 25% of the wound bed is covered with avascular tissue)
  - may have dead space
  - no signs or symptoms of infection
  - wound edges open
- *Not healing:*
  - wound with ≥25% avascular tissue (eschar and/or slough) OR
  - signs/symptoms of infection OR
  - clean but non-granulating wound bed OR
  - closed/hyperkeratotic wound edges OR
  - persistent failure to improve despite appropriate comprehensive wound management

Note: A new Stage 1 pressure ulcer is reported on OASIS as Not healing.

M0468:	**Does the patient have a Stasis Ulcer?**
M0470:	**Current number of (Observable) Stasis Ulcer(s)**
M0474:	**Does this patient have at least one Stasis Ulcer that cannot be observed?**
M0476:	**Status of the Most Problematic (Observable) Stasis Ulcer**

    1   Fully granulating
    2   Early/partial granulation
    3   Not healing
    N   No observable stasis ulcer

Definitions:

- *Fully granulating:*
  - wound bed filled with granulation tissue to the level of the surrounding skin or new epithelium
  - no dead space
  - no avascular tissue (eschar and/or slough)
  - no signs or symptoms of infection
  - wound edges are open
- *Early/partial granulation:*
  - ≥25% of the wound bed is covered with granulation tissue
  - there is minimal avascular tissue (eschar and/or slough) (i.e., < 25% of the wound bed is covered with avascular tissue)
  - may have dead space

- no signs or symptoms of infection
- wound edges open
- *Not healing:*
  - wound with ≥25% avascular tissue (eschar and/or slough) OR
  - signs/symptoms of infection OR
  - clean but non-granulating wound bed OR
  - closed/hyperkeratotic wound edges OR
  - persistent failure to improve despite appropriate comprehensive wound management

M0482: **Does the patient have a Surgical Wound?**
M0484: **Current number of (Observable) Surgical Wounds**
M0486: **Does the patient have at least one Surgical Wound that cannot be observed due to the presence of a non-removable dressing?**
M0488: **Status of the most problematic (Observable) Surgical Wound**
   1   Fully granulating
   2   Early/partial granulation
   3   Not healing
   NA   No observable surgical wound

Definitions:

- *Description/classification of wounds healing by primary intention* (i.e., approximated incisions)
  - *Fully granulating/healing:*
    - incision well-approximated with complete epithelialization of incision
    - no signs or symptoms of infection
  - *Early/partial granulation:*
    - incision well-approximated but not completely epithelialized
    - no signs or symptoms of infection
  - *Not healing:*
    - incisional separation OR
    - incisional necrosis OR
    - signs or symptoms of infection
- *Description/classification of wounds healing by secondary intention* (i.e., healing of dehisced wound by granulation, contraction and epithelialization)
  - *Fully granulating:*
    - wound bed filled with granulation tissue to the level of the surrounding skin or new epithelium
    - no dead space
    - no avascular tissue (eschar and/or slough)
    - no signs or symptoms of infection
    - wound edges are open
  - *Early/partial granulation:*
    - ≥25% of the wound bed is covered with granulation tissue
    - there is minimal avascular tissue (eschar and/or slough) (i.e., < 25% of the wound bed is covered with avascular tissue)
    - may have dead space
    - no signs or symptoms of infection
    - wound edges are open

(continues)

Exhibit 14–1 *continued*

- *Not healing:*
  - wound with ≥25% avascular tissue (eschar and/or slough) OR
  - signs/symptoms of infection OR
  - clean but non-granulating wound bed OR
  - closed/hyperkeratotic wound edges OR
  - persistent failure to improve despite comprehensive appropriate wound management

GLOSSARY

Avascular:	Lacking in blood supply; synonyms are dead, devitalized, necrotic, and nonviable. Specific types include slough and eschar.
Clean Wound:	Wound free of devitalized tissue, purulent drainage, foreign material or debris
Closed Wound Edges:	Edges of top layers of epidermis have rolled down to cover lower edge of epidermis, including basement membrane, so that epithelial cells cannot migrate from wound edges; also described as epibole. Presents clinically as sealed edge of mature epithelium; may be hard/thickened; may be discolored (e.g., yellowish, gray, or white).
Dead Space:	A defect or cavity
Dehisced/Dehiscence:	Separation of surgical incision; loss of approximation of wound edges
Epidermis:	Outermost layer of skin
Epithelialization:	Regeneration of epidermis across a wound surface
Eschar:	Black or brown necrotic, devitalized tissue; tissue can be loose or firmly adherent, hard, soft or soggy.
Full Thickness:	Tissue damage involving total loss of epidermis and dermis and extending into the subcutaneous tissue and possibly into the muscle or bone.
Granulation Tissue:	The pink/red, moist tissue comprised of new blood vessels, connective tissue, fibroblasts, and inflammatory cells, which fills an open wound when it starts to heal; typically appears deep pink or red with an irregular, "berry-like" surface
Healing:	A dynamic process involving synthesis of new tissue for repair of skin and soft tissue defects.
Hyperkeratosis:	Hard, white/gray tissue surrounding the wound
Infection:	The presence of bacteria or other microorganisms in sufficient quantity to damage tissue or impair healing. Wounds can be classified as infected when the wound tissue contains 10^5 (100,000) or greater microorganisms per gram of tissue. Typical signs and symptoms of infection include purulent exudate, odor, erythema, warmth, tenderness, edema, pain, fever, and elevated white cell count. However, clinical signs of infection may not be present, especially in theimmunocompromised patient or the patient with poor perfusion.
Necrotic Tissue:	See avascular.
Non-granulating:	Absence of granulation tissue; wound surface appears smooth as opposed to granular. For example, in a wound that is clean but non-granulating, the wound surface appears smooth and red as opposed to berry-like.

Partial Thickness:	Confined to the skin layers; damage does not penetrate below the dermis and may be limited to the epidermal layers only
Sinus Tract:	Course or path of tissue destruction occurring in any direction from the surface or edge of the wound; results in dead space with potential for abscess formation. Also sometimes called "tunneling." (Can be distinguished from undermining by fact that sinus tract involves a small portion of the wound edge whereas undermining involves a significant portion of the wound edge.)
Slough:	Soft moist avascular (devitalized) tissue; may be white, yellow, tan, or green; may be loose or firmly adherent
Tunneling:	See sinus tract
Undermining:	Area of tissue destruction extending under intact skin along the periphery of a wound; commonly seen in shear injuries. Can be distinguished from sinus tract by fact that undermining involves a significant portion of the wound edge, whereas sinus tract involves only a small portion of the wound edge.

In terms of assessing wounds, validated tools are not currently available, though progress has been made in this area. The following physical characteristics are emerging as key components of a complete wound assessment, and they should be documented initially and regularly thereafter. These include wound location, size, tissue type, exudate type and amount, and type and condition of surrounding skin. Wound assessments should also be documented regularly and with any significant change in condition, such as after a significant debridement, with increasing pain, or signs of infection. In the 2010 update, the CMS included a requirement that pressure ulcer size and depth be recorded with OASIS items M1310, M1312, and M1314. Instructions on completing OASIS items included specifics on how these measurements must be performed.

For patients with common conditions, evidence-based pathways or protocols should be developed and individualized to establish and meet the goals of the plan of care. These pathways should include specific activities and time frames to ensure each home health visit progresses the patient and family closer to the goal of stability and a maximum level of independence. Documentation should also note case conferences with regular reviews of progress and discussions of modifying the plan of care as needed. This helps maintain a realistic plan with achievable goals for the individual patient.

Wound assessment should be an integral part of the comprehensive assessment that clinicians perform and must be consistent with the OASIS data set. When documented well, they support care that is ethically sound, reimbursable, and compliant with state and federal regulations.

BIBLIOGRAPHY

CMS Home Health Care Quality Initiative. Retrieved March 25, 2011 from http://www.cms.hhs.gov/homehealthqualityinits

CMS OASIS Overview. Retrieved October 18, 2011 from https://www.cms.gov/oasis/

Leslie, C. M. (2003). The changes impacting wound care practices. *The Remington Report*, *11*(3), 14–17.

WOCN Society. Guidance on OASIS. Retrieved October 18, 2011 from http://www.wocn.org/?page=GuidanceonOASIS&hhSearchTerms=guidance

Zuber, R. (2003). Medicare survey shifts focus to outcomes. *Home Healthcare Nurse*, *3*(21), 187–191.

Pressure Ulcers in Long-Term Care

Shirley Grant
Karen Lou Kennedy-Evans
S. Kwon Lee

INTRODUCTION

Assessment and treatment of pressure ulcers in long-term care settings are no different than for acute or home care. However, in long-term care certain things need to be done on a weekly or quarterly basis or when the resident has a change in condition. The long-term care industry is heavily regulated and monitored by both the state and federal government agencies. Noncompliance with the regulations can incur heavy monetary fines and have a negative impact on new admissions to the facility until the deficiencies are corrected.

In 1987 in response to concern over the quality of care in nursing homes, Congress directed Health Care Financing Administration (HCFA), now the Centers for Medicare and Medicaid Services (CMS), to study ways to improve the quality of nursing home care. Legislation to improve the quality of care in nursing homes was enacted and became known as the Omnibus Budget Reconciliation Act (OBRA). The OBRA regulations mandate patient assessment, limit psychotropic drug use, and ensure residents' rights.

The regulations by CMS governing nursing homes are called F-tags. The F-tag pertaining to pressure ulcers is called F314. This regulation, including enforcement guidelines, is approximately 25 pages long (*The Facility Guide*, 2010).

F314 states: Based on a comprehensive assessment of a resident, the facility must ensure that:

(1) A resident who enters the facility without pressure sores does not develop pressure sores unless the individual's clinical condition demonstrates that they were unavoidable; and

(2) A resident having pressure sores receives necessary treatment and services to promote healing, prevent infection and prevent new sores from developing.

This chapter discusses the following areas pertaining to pressure ulcers in long-term care: risk assessment and documentation, care planning, prevention, and management.

RISK ASSESSMENT AND DOCUMENTATION

When an individual is admitted into a long-term care facility three issues must be addressed:

1. The overall patient assessment, which includes an initial skin assessment.
2. A risk assessment for pressure ulcers.
3. The initial Resident Assessment Instrument (RAI), which includes the Minimum Data Set (MDS), Care Area Assessments (CAAs), formerly the Resident Assessment Protocols (RAPs), and the resident's care plan.

Once the admission skin assessment and pressure ulcer risk assessment are completed, it is appropriate to initiate a temporary care plan. It is recommended that evaluating the skin condition be done on a weekly basis. Evaluation can include such factors as color, moisture, temperature, integrity, and turgor. It also is recommended that a standardized pressure ulcer risk assessment tool be used to assess a resident's pressure ulcer risk upon admission, weekly for the first 4 weeks after admission for each resident at risk, then quarterly, or whenever there is a change in condition or change of functional ability. If a resident has a pressure ulcer, the weekly pressure ulcer assessments should be done. Three items must be completed no less than quarterly: (1) MDS Item Set, (2) Quarterly Pressure Ulcer Risk Assessment, and (3) Care Plan review and revision. The areas that need to be assessed or monitored daily, weekly, quarterly, or with a change in the resident's condition are discussed in more detail later in this chapter.

Pressure Ulcer Risk Evaluation/Assessment

When an individual is admitted to a long-term care facility a pressure ulcer risk assessment needs to be done to determine if the resident is at risk for developing pressure ulcers. This can be done with a validated assessment tool such as the Braden or the Norton Scale. However, the only mandated assessment tool according to F314 is the RAI (CMS, 2010). The "at-risk assessment" may be done by a Licensed Practical/Vocational Nurse (LP/VN) where state statutes permit and according to individual facility policy. If the resident is at risk for pressure ulcers the preventative measures implemented should be included as a part of the care plan. The "at-risk assessment" is recommended to be done upon admission, weekly for 4 weeks (total of 5 times) then quarterly.

Risk factors for pressure ulcers can be many. Those mentioned in F314 are not limited to impaired/decreased mobility and decreased functional ability; co-morbid conditions, such as end stage renal disease, thyroid disease or diabetes mellitus; drugs such as steroids that may affect wound healing; impaired diffuse or localized blood flow, such as generalized atherosclerosis or lower extremity arterial insufficiency; resident refusal of some aspects of care and treatment:

cognitive impairment; exposure of skin to urinary and fecal incontinence; under nutrition, malnutrition, and hydration deficits; and a healed ulcer.

Risk factors can be defined as anything that increases the chance of developing a pressure ulcer. (Wound, Ostomy, and Continence Nursing [WOCN] Society, 2010). More than 100 risk factors have been reported in the literature to be associated with pressure ulcer development (Lyder & Ayello, 2008).

When the Braden Scale is used, if major risk factors such as age, fever, poor dietary intake of protein, diastolic pressure < 60 and/or hemodynamic instability are present, advance to the next level of risk (Ayello & Braden, 2002). The Minimum Data Set (MDS) 3.0 also states an individual is at risk for pressure ulcers if they have a Stage I pressure ulcer or greater, a scar over a bony prominence, or a nonremovable dressing or device. If a nonremovable dressing or device is in place, it is important to monitor the surrounding skin for signs of redness, swelling, increased drainage, or tenderness to touch, and adequate pain control.

Minimum Data Set 3.0

The MDS 3.0 became effective October 1, 2010. Section M of the MDS 3.0 is devoted entirely to skin and pressure ulcers. This document needs to be completed on admission (within the first 14 days), quarterly, and when the resident experiences a change of condition. Additional MDS assessments may be required by resident circumstances, regulatory agencies or payor sources. Treatments for pressure ulcers mentioned on the MDS 3.0 are: pressure reducing device for chair/bed, turning/repositioning program, nutritional or hydration intervention and ulcer care.

Photo Documentation

Photo documentation may be used to support written or electronic documentation. The facility should develop a protocol consistent with accepted standards such as frequency of photo documentation, consistent distance from the wound, type of equipment used, and means to ensure digital images are accurate and not modified. F314 recommends including within the photo image the resident identification, ulcer location, and date. HIPAA (Health Insurance Portability and Accountability Act) regulations specify there should not be any identifying characteristics in the picture such as name, initials, date, birthdate, Social Security number, patient ID number, or tattoos.

CARE PLANNING

The care plan for a resident at risk for developing a pressure ulcer or a resident who has a pressure ulcer should include prevention, care, and treatment of the pressure ulcer. Care plans are composed of a statement of the issue(s) identified, goals/measurable objectives with approximate time frames, and interventions. Care plans are to be completed on admission, quarterly, when a pressure ulcer is healed, when changes are identified in risk factors or treatment regimens, and when the current treatment approach is ineffective.

Although preventive measures are much the same for the majority of residents, the best way to ensure an individualized plan of care is to update the care plan when the treatment is changed. This can be done simply by adding "Treatment changed" and the date the treatment was changed to the care plan. It is not necessary to specify the details of the actual treatment change. Items to consider including on the care plan for prevention and treatment include repositioning, floating the heels, skin care for incontinence, support surfaces, and maintaining or improving nutrition/hydration. Efforts should be made to stabilize, reduce, or remove underlying risk factors and to monitor the impact of the interventions and modify them as appropriate based on the individual needs of the resident.

PRESSURE ULCER PREVENTION

Pressure-Reducing Device for the Bed

According to the WOCN (2010) Guidelines, pressure redistribution surfaces are recommended for individuals with full-thickness (stage III or IV) ulcers or ulcers that involve multiple turning surfaces. For patients with large stage III or IV pressure ulcers or ulcers on multiple turning surfaces, a low air-loss or air-fluidized surface may be indicated. Mackey (2005) states, "Based on the current research it is impossible to determine the most effective support surface for the treatment of pressure ulcers."

According to the National Pressure Ulcer Advisory Panel, the terms "pressure reducing" and "pressure reduction" have been replaced with "pressure redistribution."

Pressure-Reducing Device for the Chair According to the WOCN (2010) Guidelines, chair cushions have not been adequately evaluated to allow recommending one over another (McInnes, et al., 2008).

Turning/Repositioning Program

Residents dependent on staff for repositioning may benefit from repositioning every 2 hours or more frequently depending on the resident's individual risk factors and tissue tolerance. According to the American Medical Directors Association (AMDA, 2008) tissue tolerance is the ability of the skin and its supporting structures to endure the effects of pressure without adverse effects. Tissue tolerance varies among individuals.

Nutrition or Hydration Intervention

There are no wound-specific nutritional measures. Unless contraindicated, nutritional goals for a resident with nutritional compromise who has a pressure ulcer or is at risk of developing pressure ulcers should include protein intake of approximately 1.2–1.5 gm/kg body weight daily (higher end of the range for those with larger, more extensive, or multiple wounds.) A simple multivitamin is appropriate, but unless the resident has a specific vitamin or mineral deficiency, supplementation with additional vitamins or minerals may not be indicated.

Labs

To help establish overall prognosis, a serum albumin, prealbumin, and cholesterol test may be useful; however, it may not correlate well with clinical observation of nutritional status. At his or her discretion, a practitioner may order test(s) that provide additional information or help with management of treatable conditions. A low albumin along with a facility's lack of supplementation, for example, is not sufficient to site a pressure ulcer deficiency according to F314.

PRESSURE ULCER MANAGEMENT AND TREATMENT

When a new pressure ulcer is identified, the following steps should be taken:

1. Assess the pressure ulcer.
2. Notify the physician or primary care practitioner and obtain a treatment order for the pressure ulcer.
3. Notify the patient, family, or responsible party.
4. Add the pressure ulcer to the care plan.
5. Assess the risk factors and modify these on the care plan as needed.
6. Add the pressure ulcer to the facility's pressure ulcer list.

Pressure Ulcer Assessment

If the patient develops a pressure ulcer, F314 suggests that the following characteristics be included in the pressure ulcer assessment:

- name
- date
- location
- stage
- size (perpendicular measurements of the greatest extent of length and width of the ulceration)
- depth (from visible surface to deepest area)

- sinus tract
- tunneling
- undermining
- necrotic tissue
- slough
- eschar
- exudate (such as serous or purulent)
- drainage odor
- drainage approximate amount
- pain, if present whether episodic or continuous
- evidence of healing (granulation tissue) or necrosis (slough or eschar)
- description of wound edges (rolled edges) and surrounding tissue (redness, hardness or induration or maceration) as appropriate

It is important for documentation in the resident's medical record to reflect the findings of each assessment.

The MDS 3.0 considers the pressure ulcer length as the longest length from head to toe and width as the widest width of the same pressure ulcer, side-to-side perpendicular (90-degree angle) to length.

Exudate amounts vary with each wound. Minimum amount might be < 5 cc in 24 hours and one gauze change per day, moderate, 5–10 cc in 24 hours and 2–3 gauze changes per day and high, >10 cc in 24 hours and 3 or more gauze changes per day.

Reassessment

F314 states, "If a pressure ulcer fails to show some evidence of progress toward healing within 2–4 weeks, the pressure ulcer (including potential complications) and the resident's overall clinical condition should be reassessed."

The WOCN (2010) Guidelines recommend that if a reduction in wound volume is not noted in 4 to 6 weeks, reevaluate the wound and revise the treatment plan as indicated. Parameters to assess healing include wound dimensions, exudate, and tissue type.

Ulcer Care

F314 states that no particular dressing promotes healing of all pressure ulcers within an ulcer classification.

Avoidable/Unavoidable Pressure Ulcers

In long-term care there are distinctions to determine if a pressure ulcer is avoidable or unavoidable. F314 explains the difference between avoidable and unavoidable:

Avoidable

The resident developed a pressure ulcer and the facility **did not** do one of the following: Evaluate the resident's clinical condition and pressure ulcer risk factors; define and implement interventions that are consistent with resident needs, resident goals, and recognized standards of practice; monitor and evaluate the impact of the interventions; or revise the interventions as appropriate.

Unavoidable

The resident developed a pressure ulcer **even though** the facility had evaluated the resident's clinical condition and pressure ulcer risk factors; defined and implemented interventions that are consistent with resident's needs, goals, and recognized standards of practice; monitored and evaluated the impact of the interventions; and revised the approaches as appropriate.

Unavoidable in F314 might be identified during the admission evaluation by the presence of preexisting signs (such as a purple or very dark area that is surrounded by profound redness, edema, or induration) suggesting that deep tissue damage has already occurred and additional deep tissue loss may occur. This deep tissue damage could lead to the appearance of an unavoidable Stage III or IV pressure ulcer or progression of a Stage I pressure ulcer to an ulcer with eschar or exudate within days after admission.

The AMDA (2008) clinical practice guideline section on unavoidable pressure ulcers describes a retrospective review of data collected over a 5-year period in a 500-bed intermediate-care facility, in which Kennedy described an ulcer with specific characteristics that was observed in patients close to death. The "Kennedy Terminal Ulcer" is described as usually appearing on the sacrum and as generally having a sudden onset and rapid progressions. Initially, it may resemble an abrasion, black spot or small blister; it quickly deepens and changes color (from red to yellow to black). Some terminally ill patients developed ulcers with these characteristics.

Skin Issues Confused with Pressure Ulcers

Stage I and II pressure ulcers can be confused with Incontinent Associated Dermatitis (IAD) and/or Moisture Associated Skin Damage (MASD). IAD and MASD usually present as a localized area of erythema, scaling, itching, papules, weeping, and eruptions or skin discoloration. It is a more diffuse area of erythema or discoloration where urine and stool come in contact with the skin. Skin tears are also not considered pressure ulcers.

Refusal of Care

If a resident chooses to exercise his or her right to make informed choices about care and treatment or to refuse treatment, the facility and the resident (or the resident's legal representative) must discuss the resident's condition, treatment options, expected outcomes, and consequences of refusing treatment. It is important to document these discussions in the resident's medical record.

Do Not Resuscitate

The presence of a "Do Not Resuscitate" (DNR) order is not sufficient to indicate that the resident is declining other appropriate treatment and services. It indicates only that the resident has chosen not to be resuscitated if respirations and/or cardiac function ceases according to F314.

Medical Director's Responsibility

A facility should be able to show that its treatment protocols are based upon current standards of practice and are in accord with the facility's policies and procedures as developed with the medical director's review and approval according to F314.

REFERENCES

Agency for Health Care Policy and Research. (1994). *Treatment of pressure ulcers.* Quick Reference Guideline Number 15, Washington, DC: U.S. Department of Health and Human Services, Public Health Service, Agency for Health Care Policy and Research.

American Medical Directors Association. (2008). *Pressure ulcers in the long-term care setting.* Clinical Practice Guideline. Columbia, MD: Author.

Ayello, E. A., & Braden, B. (2002), How and why to do pressure ulcer assessment. *Advances in Skin and Wound Care, 15*(3), 125–131.

Centers for Medicare and Medicaid Services (CMS). (2010). Long-term care facility Resident Assessment Instrument user's manual (Version 3.0), Washington, DC: U.S. Department of Health and Human Services.

Krasner, D. L., Rodeheaver, G. T., & Sibbald, R. G. (2007). *Chronic wound care:* A *clinical source book for healthcare professionals* (4th ed.). Malvern, PA: HMP Communications.

Lyder & Ayello, (2008)

Mackey, (2005)

McInnes, et al., (2008)

The facility guide to OBRA regulations and the long term care survey process. (2010). Miamisburg, OH: MED-PASS. (Rev. 70, Issued: 01-07-11, effective: 10/01/10, Implementation: 10-01-10)

Wound, Ostomy and Continence Nurses Society, (2010). *Guideline for prevention and management of pressure ulcers,* Mount Laurel, NJ: Author.

You Are Not Alone in Wound Care

Jo A. Patterson

Caregivers, patients, and at times nurses and clinicians can feel isolated as they try to find help in caring for patients with wounds. Here is great news! You are not alone. There are excellent resources, associations, and educational opportunities available to you. In most cases the resources are free of charge. So go online, explore, download, and research what you need. Take advantage of what is available so you can give better care for your patients and facilitate wound healing.

The following is a list of websites offering CEUs, a list of professional organizations, and free information online about caring for patients with wounds.

FREE CEUs/LIBRARY SOURCES

The Wound Institute

http://www.thewoundinstitute.com
   The Wound Institute by Healthpoint offers comprehensive, interactive wound care courses. All courses are offered at no cost to clinicians, are fully continuing education/continuing medical education (CE/CME) accredited, and are available 24/7.

Medscape Nurses Homepage

http://www.medscape.com/nurses
   The Medscape Nurses homepage is a library of everything needed for the advanced and specialty nursing practice.

North American Center for Continuing Medical Education (NACCME)

www.naccme.com
   NACCME's website is a full-service division offering educational programs to a wide rage of clients in the healthcare profession.

Smith & Nephew—The Global Wound Academy

www.globalwoundacademy.com
  The Smith & Nephew wound management site, the Global Wound Academy, has been developed to provide worldwide access to education and information about the therapeutic area of wound management.

KCI Wound Vacuum

www.kci1.com
  KCI's wound care education programs are designed to support and provide information to clinicians on wound types, assessment, care planning, interventions, products, and outcomes management.

PROFESSIONAL ORGANIZATIONS AND WEBSITES

Association for the Advancement of Wound Care (AAWC)

www.aawconline.org
  AAWC is a nonprofit organization dedicated to the multidisciplinary approach to wound care. Membership is open to all individuals, facilities, corporations, lay caregivers, patients, and others interested in wound care. AAWC exists to build a collaborative community to facilitate optimal care for those who suffer with wounds.
  The AAWC official journals are *Ostomy Wound Management* (OWM), www.o-wm.com; WOUNDS A *Compendium of Clinical Research and Practice*, www.woundsresearch.com.

American Academy of Wound Management (AAWM)

www.aawm.org
  The American Academy of Wound Management is a voluntary, not-for-profit organization established for the purpose of credentialing interdisciplinary practitioners in wound management. The purpose of the American Academy of Wound Management is to establish and administer a certification process in wound management. The American Academy of Wound Management has administered its Certified Wound Specialist (CWS) examination to more than 1,500 multidisciplinary professionals over the past 5 years. CWS has emerged as the predominant interdisciplinary certification in wound care. A Certified Wound Care Associate (CWCA) program is also available.

The American College of Certified Wound Specialists™ (ACCWS)

www.theccws.org
  Composed of interdisciplinary wound care professionals, the American College of Certified Wound Specialists promotes awareness and understanding of the potential impact the Certified Wound Specialist® (CWS®) can have on general health care.

American Professional Wound Care Association (APWCA)

www.apwca.org

The American Professional Wound Care Association is a hybrid nonprofit organization unlike any other organization available. The APWCA is a membership organization incorporating the various medical specialties involved in treating complex wounds. Our seminars bring these fields together and therefore facilitate an integrated, multidisciplinary approach. The mission of the association is to help decrease the rate of complications from all wounds, including acute, chronic, postsurgical, postradiation, reconstructive, and other problematic wounds. Their goal is to accelerate wound healing and preserve and/or enhance the quality of life for these patients. This broad definition reflecting interest in all forms of wounds is one factor that distinguishes APWCA from other organizations and associations in wound care. APWCA's endorsed journal is *Advances in Skin & Wound Care*, the Journal for Prevention and Healing, www.woundcarejournal.com.

Baromedical Nurses Association (BNA)

www.hyperbaricnurses.org

The BNA provides nurses with a professional organization to maintain and promote the status and standards of practice in hyperbaric nursing.

Undersea & Hyperbaric Medical Society (UHMS)

www.uhms.org

The UHMS is an international, not-for-profit organization serving over 2,500 members from more than 50 countries. Most UHMS members are diving or hyperbaric scientists and physicians. The associate members are composed of nurses, technicians, respiratory therapists, and others who work in the field of diving and hyperbaric medicine. The Undersea & Hyperbaric Medical Society (UHMS) is the primary source of information for diving and hyperbaric medicine physiology worldwide. It was founded as the Undersea Medical Society in 1967, but in 1986 it changed the name to Undersea & Hyperbaric Medical Society. The name change reflects the rapidly growing interest in hyperbaric oxygen physiology and therapy. The UHMS's purpose is to provide scientific information to protect the health of sport, military, and commercial divers and to improve the scientific basis of hyperbaric oxygen therapy, promote sound treatment protocols and standards of practice, and provide CME accreditation.

National Board of Diving and Hyperbaric Medical Technology (NBDHMT)

www.nbdhmt.org

The mission of the National Board of Diving and Hyperbaric Medical Technology is to provide board certification and ongoing support to hyperbaric technologists, hyperbaric nurses, and diving medical technicians to ensure that the fields of hyperbaric medicine and hyperbaric chamber operation are staffed with the most highly qualified personnel as possible.

Best Publishing Company

www.bestpub.com

Best Publishing Company is one of the largest publishers of diving, underwater, and hyperbaric medicine books in the world. The *Hyperbaric Medicine Product and Resource Guide* is available at www.HyperbaricGuide.com.

Canadian Association of Wound Care (CAWC)

www.cawc.net

The CAWC is a nonprofit organization of healthcare professionals, industry participants, patients, and caregivers dedicated to the advancement of wound care in Canada.

Wound, Ostomy, and Continence Nurses Society (WOCN)

www.wocn.org

The Wound, Ostomy, and Continence Nurses Society is a professional, international nursing society of more than 4,000 nurse professionals who are experts in the care of patients with wound, ostomy, and continence problems.

Wound, Ostomy, and Continence Nursing Certification Board (WOCNCB)

www.wocncb.org

The Wound, Ostomy, and Continence Nursing Certification Board (WOCNCB) is a professional organization dedicated to promoting the highest standard of consumer care and safety by providing credentialing in the areas of wound, ostomy, continence, and foot care nursing. The credentials offered are CWOCN®, CWCN®, COCN®, CWON™, CCCN®, and CFCN®.

Information has been reproduced with permission from individual organizations.

Abscess. A circumscribed collection of pus that forms in tissue as a result of acute or chronic localized infection. It is associated with tissue destruction and frequently swelling.

Acute Wounds. Disruptions in the skin integrity and underlying tissues that progress through the healing process in a timely manner without complications.

Adherent Materials. Matter attached to the wound bed such as eschar, dirt particles, or bacteria.

Albumin. A major plasma protein. Numerous studies have revealed increased morbidity and mortality in patients with decreased serum albumin levels. The normal serum albumin concentration is 3.5 to 5.0 gm/dL. This value is effective showing nutritional status 3–4 weeks prior to lab draw. (See Hypoalbuminemia)

Ankle-Brachial Index. Doppler-derived lower extremity arterial pressures are measured and an ankle-brachial index (ABI) is calculated by making a ratio of pressure at the ankle to pressure in the arm. The normal ABI is 0.9 to 1.1.

Antiseptic (Topical). Product with antimicrobial activity designed for use on skin or other superficial tissues; may damage cells.

Arterial Ulcer. Wounds that are caused by insufficient arterial perfusion. These wounds are usually painful. Clinically, they may appear as "punched out" wounds that have pale wound beds, well-defined wound edges, and minimal exudate.

Atherosclerosis. Plaque formation on the walls of arteries causing a narrowing of the lumen and decreased blood flow.

Avascular. Lacking in blood supply; synonyms are dead, devitalized, necrotic, and nonviable. Specific types include slough and eschar.

Bottoming Out. Expression used to describe inadequate support from a mattress overlay or seat cushion as determined by a "hand check." To perform a hand check, the caregiver places an outstretched hand (palm up) under the overlay or cushion below the pressure ulcer or that part of the body at risk for a pressure ulcer. If the caregiver feels less than an inch of support material, the patient has bottomed out and the support surface is therefore inadequate.

Cellulitis. Inflammation of cellular or connective tissue. Inflammation may be diminished or absent in immunosuppressed individuals.

Cellulitis (Advancing). Cellulitis that is visibly spreading in the area of the wound. Advancement can be monitored by marking the outer edge of the cellulitis and assessing the area for advancement or spread 24 hours later.

Chronic Wounds. These nonhealing wounds deviate from the expected sequence of repair in terms of time, appearance, and response to appropriate treatments.

Clean. Containing no foreign material or debris.

Clean Dressing. Dressing that is not sterile but is free of environmental contaminants such as water damage, dust, pest and rodent contaminants, and gross soiling.

Clean Wound. Wound free of purulent drainage, devitalized tissue, or dirt.

Closed Wound Edges. Edges of top layers of epidermis have rolled down to cover lower edge of epidermis, including basement membrane, so that epithelial cells cannot migrate from wound edges; Also described as epibole or hyperkeratotic. Presents clinically as sealed edge of mature epithelium; and wound edge may present clinically as hard/thickened; and/or discolored (e.g., yellowish, gray, or white).

Colonized. The presence of bacteria on the surface or in the tissue of a wound without indications of infection, such as purulent exudate, foul odor, or surrounding inflammation. All Stage II, III, and IV pressure ulcers are colonized.

Contaminated. Containing bacteria, other microorganisms, or foreign material. The term usually refers to bacterial contamination and in this context is synonymous with colonized. Wounds with bacterial counts of 10^5 organisms per gram of tissue or less are generally considered to be contaminated; those with higher counts are generally considered to be infected.

Culture and Sensitivity. Removal of bacteria from a wound for the purpose of placing them in a growth medium in the laboratory to propagate to the point where they can be identified and tested for sensitivity to various antibiotics.

Culture (Swab). Technique involving the use of a swab to remove bacteria from a wound and placing them in a growth medium for propagation and identification. Swab cultures obtained from the surface of a pressure ulcer are usually positive because of surface colonization and should not be used to diagnose ulcer infection.

Dead Space. A cavity remaining in a wound.

Debridement. Removal of devitalized tissue and foreign matter from a wound. Various methods can be used for this purpose:

Autolytic Debridement. The use of synthetic dressings to cover a wound and allow eschar to self-digest by the action of enzymes present in wound fluids.

Enzymatic (Chemical) Debridement. The topical application of proteolytic substances (enzymes) to break down devitalized tissue.

Mechanical Debridement. Removal of foreign material and devitalized or contaminated tissue from a wound by physical forces rather than by chemical (enzymatic) or natural (autolytic) forces. Examples are wet-to-dry dressings, wound irrigation, whirlpool, and dextranomers.

Sharp Debridement. Removal of foreign material or devitalized tissue by a sharp instrument such as a scalpel. Laser debridement is also considered to be a type of sharp debridement.

Dehisced/Dehiscence. Separation of the layers of a surgical wound. Separation of surgical incision; loss of approximation of wound edges.

Dermis. Inner layer of skin that contains the hair follicles and sweat glands. A Stage II pressure ulcer will involve this layer of skin.

Deterioration. Negative course. Failure of the pressure ulcer to heal, as shown by wound enlargement that is not brought about by debridement.

Dextranomers. Highly hydrophilic dextran-polymer beads that are poured into secreting wounds to absorb wound exudates and act as a debriding agent.

Dressing. The material applied to a wound for the protection of the wound and absorbance of drainage.

> **Alginate Dressing.** A nonwoven, absorptive dressing manufactured from seaweed.
>
> **Film Dressing.** A clear, adherent, nonabsorptive, polymer-based dressing that is permeable to oxygen and water vapor but not to water.
>
> **Foam Dressing.** A spongelike polymer dressing that may or may not be adherent; it may be impregnated or coated with other materials and has some absorptive properties.
>
> **Gauze Dressing.** A cotton or synthetic fabric dressing that is absorptive and permeable to water, water vapor, and oxygen. This dressing may be impregnated with petrolatum, antiseptics, or other agents.
>
>> **Continuously Moist Saline Gauze.** A dressing technique in which gauze moistened with normal saline is applied to the wound and remoistened frequently enough so it will remain moist. The goal is to maintain a continuously moist wound environment.
>>
>> **Wet-to-Dry Saline Gauze.** A dressing technique in which gauze moistened with normal saline is applied wet to the wound and removed once the gauze becomes dry and adheres to the wound bed. The goal is to debride the wound as the dressing is removed.
>
> **Hydrocolloid Dressing.** An adhesive, moldable wafer made of a carbohydrate-based material, usually with a waterproof backing. This dressing usually is impermeable to oxygen, water, and water vapor and has some absorptive properties.
>
> **Hydrogel Dressing.** A water-based, nonadherent, polymer-based dressing that has some absorptive properties.
>
> **Pastes/Powders/Beads.** Agents formulated primarily to fill wound cavities that may have some absorptive properties.

Epidermis. Avascular outer layer of the skin. New epidermis appears pink and dry and may look shiny.

Epithelialization. The stage of tissue healing in which the epithelial cells migrate (move) across the surface of a wound. During this stage of healing, the epithelium appears the color of "ground glass" to pink.

Erythema. Redness of the skin.

    Blanchable Erythema. Reddened area that temporarily turns white or pale when pressure is applied with a fingertip. Blanchable erythema over a pressure site is usually due to a normal reactive hyperemic response.

    Nonblanchable Erythema. Redness that persists when fingertip pressure is applied. Nonblanchable erythema over a pressure site is a symptom of a Stage I pressure ulcer.

Eschar. Thick, leathery, necrotic, devitalized tissue; can be loose or firmly adherent, hard, soft, dry, or wet.

Exudate. Any fluid that has been extruded from a tissue or its capillaries, more specifically because of injury or inflammation. It is characteristically high in protein and white blood cells.

Fascia. A sheet or band of fibrous tissue that lies deep below the skin or encloses muscles and various organs of the body.

Fluid Irrigation. Cleansing by means of a stream of fluid, preferably saline.

Friction. Mechanical force exerted when skin is dragged across a coarse surface such as bed linens.

Full-Thickness Tissue Loss. Tissue damage involving total loss of epidermis and dermis and extending into the subcutaneous tissue and possibly into the muscle or bone.

Granulation Tissue. The pink/red, moist tissue that contains new blood vessels, collagen, fibroblasts, and inflammatory cells, which fills an open, previously deep wound when it starts to heal.

Growth Factors. Proteins that affect the proliferation, movement, maturation, and biosynthetic activity of cells. For the purposes of this guideline, these are proteins that can be produced by living cells.

Handwashing. Handwashing is the cornerstone of any infection-control program. Handwashing should be of sufficient duration to remove the transient microbial flora (10 seconds of soap and friction, followed by rinsing with running water).

Healing. A dynamic process in which anatomical and functional integrity is restored. This process can be monitored and measured. For wounds of the skin, it involves repair of the dermis (granulation tissue formation) and epidermis (epithelialization). Healed wounds represent a spectrum of repair: They can be ideally healed (tissue regeneration), minimally healed (temporary return of anatomical continuity), or acceptably healed (sustained functional and anatomical result). The acceptably healed wound is the ultimate outcome of wound healing but not necessarily the appropriate outcome for all patients.

Primary Intention Healing. Closure and healing of a sutured wound.

Secondary Intention Healing. Closure and healing of a wound by the formation of granulation tissue and epithelialization.

Hydrotherapy. Use of whirlpool or submersion for wound cleansing.

Hyperkeratosis. Hard, white/gray tissue surrounding a wound.

Hypoalbuminemia. An abnormally low amount of albumin in the blood. A value less than 3.5 mg/dL is clinically significant. Albumin is the major serum protein that maintains plasma colloidal osmotic pressure (pressure within blood vessels) and transports fatty acids, bilirubin, and many drugs as well as certain hormones, such as cortisol and thyroxine, through the blood. Low serum albumin may be due to inadequate protein intake, active inflammation, or serious hepatic and renal disease and is associated with pressure ulcer development.

Infection. The presence of bacteria or other microorganisms in sufficient quantity to damage tissue or impair healing. Clinical experience has indicated that wounds can be classified as infected when the wound tissue contains 10^5 or more microorganisms per gram of tissue. Clinical signs of infection may not be present, especially in the immunocompromised patient or the patient with a chronic wound.

Infection (Clinical). The presence of bacteria or other microorganisms in sufficient quantity to overwhelm the tissue defenses and produce the inflammatory signs of infection (i.e., purulent exudate, odor, erythema, warmth, tenderness, edema, pain, fever, and elevated white cell count).

Local Clinical Infection. A clinical infection that is confined to the wound and within a few millimeters of its margins.

Systemic Clinical Infection. A clinical infection that extends beyond the margins of the wound. Some systemic infectious complications of pressure ulcers include cellulitis, advancing cellulitis, osteomyelitis, meningitis, endocarditis, septic arthritis, bacteremia, and sepsis.

Inflammatory Response. A localized protective response elicited by injury or destruction of tissues that serves to destroy, dilute, or wall off both the injurious agent and the injured tissue. Clinical signs include pain, heat, redness, swelling, and loss of function. Inflammation may be diminished or absent in immunosuppressed patients.

Innervation. Nerve supply to an area of the body. Innervation is considered to be adequate if it is sufficient to sense temperature, touch, and pressure/pain and communicate this sensory information to the brain.

Intention. See Healing.

Irrigation. Cleansing by a stream of fluid, preferably saline.

Ischemia. Deficiency of blood supply to a tissue, often leading to tissue necrosis.

Macerate. To soften by wetting or soaking. In this context, it refers to degenerative changes and disintegration of skin when it has been kept too moist.

Malnutrition. State of nutritional insufficiency due to either inadequate dietary intake or defective assimilation or utilization of ingested food. Clinically significant malnutrition is diagnosed if (1) serum albumin is less than 3.5 mg/dL, (2) the total lymphocyte count is less than 1800/mm^3, or (3) body weight has decreased more than 15%.

Necrotic Tissue. Tissue that has died and has therefore lost its usual physical properties and biological activity. Also called "devitalized tissue."

Newly Epithelialized. The process of regeneration of the epidermis across a wound surface or regeneration of the epidermis across a wound surface.

Nonepithelialized. The absence of regenerated epidermis across a wound surface.

Nongranulating. Absence of granulation tissue; wound surface appears smooth as opposed to granular. For example, in a wound that is clean but non-granulating, the wound surface appears smooth and red as opposed to berry-like.

No-Touch Technique. Method of changing surface dressings without touching the wound or the surface of any dressing that may be in contact with the wound. Adherent dressings should be grasped by the corner and removed slowly, whereas gauze dressings can be pinched in the center and lifted off.

Osteomyelitis. An infectious inflammatory disease process in the bone that is often bacterial. One cost-effective method to determine osteomyelitis is to probe the wound with a sterile cotton-tipped application. If the tip can touch bone, osteomyelitis will be present in as many as 85% of the cases.

Pain. Nerve endings exposed to dressing removal and air can cause patients extreme discomfort. Moist wound healing is highly successful at reducing pain related to trauma of dressing removal.

Partial-Thickness Tissue Loss. Wounds that involve the epidermis and can extend into, but not through, the dermis. These wounds heal mainly by epithelialization, from the wound edges and from epithelial cells in the remaining hair follicles and glands.

Periwound. The area surrounding the wound. Assessment of the edges may help to identify undermining (blue-gray or blanched), infection (erythema), or maceration (white margins).

Pressure (Interface). Force per unit area that acts perpendicularly to the body from the support surface. This parameter is affected by the stiffness of the support surface, the composition of the body tissue, and the geometry of the body being supported.

Pressure Reduction. Reduction of interface pressure, not necessarily below the level required to close capillaries (i.e., capillary-closing pressure).

Pressure Relief. Reduction of interface pressure below capillary-closing pressure.

Pressure Ulcer. Any lesion caused by unrelieved pressure resulting in damage of underlying tissue. They are also called decubitus ulcers, pressure sores, or bedsores. They are usually located over bony prominences and are graded or staged to classify the degree of tissue damage observed.

psi. Pounds per square inch—a unit of pressure; in this case, the pressure exerted by a stream of fluid against 1 square inch of skin or wound surface.

Purulent Discharge/Drainage. A product of inflammation that contains pus— i.e., cells (leukocytes, bacteria) and liquefied necrotic debris.

Reactive Hyperemia. Reddening of the skin caused by blood rushing back into ischemic tissue.

Repositioning. Any change in body position that relieves pressure from tissue overlying bony prominences. Periodic repositioning of chairbound and bedfast individuals is one of the most basic and frequently used methods of reducing pressure. The overall goal of repositioning is to allow tissue reperfusion and thus prevent ischemic tissue changes. The term "repositioning" implies a sustained relief of pressure, not just a temporary shift. Specific repositioning techniques and the frequency of repositioning should be individualized according to the patient's level of risk and the goals of care.

Scab. A crust of dried blood and serum.

Sepsis. The presence of various pus-forming and other pathogenic organisms or their toxins in the blood or tissues. Clinical signs of bloodborne sepsis include fever, tachycardia, hypotension, leukocytosis, and a deterioration in mental status. The same organism is often isolated in both the blood and the pressure ulcer.

Shear. Mechanical force that acts on a unit area of skin in a direction parallel to the body's surface. Shear is affected by the amount of pressure exerted, the coefficient of friction between the materials contacting each other, and the extent to which the body makes contact with the support surface.

Sinus Tract. A cavity or channel underlying a wound that involves an area larger than the visible surface of the wound. Course or path of tissue destruction occurring in any direction from the surface or edge of the wound; results in dead space with potential for abscess formation. Also sometimes called "tunneling." (Can be distinguished from undermining by the fact that the sinus tract involves a small portion of the wound edge whereas undermining involves a significant portion of the wound edge.)

Slough. Necrotic (dead) tissue in the process of separating from viable portions of the body. Soft moist avascular (devitalized) tissue; may be white, yellow, tan, grey, or green; may be loose or firmly adherent.

Stasis Ulcer. Ulceration associated with ambulatory venous hypertension.

Support Surfaces. Special beds, mattresses, mattress overlays, or seat cushions that reduce or relieve pressure while sitting or lying.

Surfactants. A surface-active agent that reduces the surface tension of fluids to allow greater penetration.

Topical Antibiotic. A drug known to inhibit or kill microorganisms that can be applied locally to a tissue surface.

Topical Antiseptic. Product with antimicrobial activity designed for use on skin or other superficial tissues; may damage some cells.

Trochanter. Bony prominence on the upper part of the femur.

Tunneling. A passageway under the surface of the skin that is generally open at the skin level; however, most of the tunneling is not visible. See sinus tract.

Underlying Tissue. Tissue that lies beneath the surface of the skin, such as fatty tissue, supporting structures, muscle, and bone.

Undermining. A closed passageway under the surface of the skin that is open only at the skin surface. Generally it appears as an area of skin ulceration at the margins of the ulcer with skin overlying the area. Undermining often develops from shearing forces. Can be distinguished from the sinus tract by the fact that undermining involves a significant portion of the wound edge, whereas sinus tract involves only a small portion of the wound edge.

Unhealed. The absence of the skin's original integrity.

Quick Assessment
of Leg Ulcers

	Venous Insufficiency (Stasis)	Arterial Insufficiency	Peripheral Neuropathy
History	Previous DVT and varicosities Reduced mobility Obesity Vascular ulcers Phlebitis Traumatic injury CHF Orthopaedic procedures Pain reduced by elevation	Diabetes Anemia Arthritis Increased pain with activity and/or elevation CVA Smoking Intermittent claudication Traumatic injury to extremity Vascular procedures/ surgeries Hypertension Hyperlipidemia Arterial disease	Diabetes Spinal cord injury Hansen's disease Relief of pain with ambulation Paresthesia of extremities
Location	Medial aspect of lower leg and ankle Superior to medial malleolus	Toe tips or web spaces Phalangeal heads around lateral malleolus Areas exposed to pressure or repetitive trauma	Plantar aspect of foot Metatarsal heads Heels Altered pressure points/sites of painless trauma/ repetitive stress
Appearance	Color: base ruddy Surrounding skin: erythema (venous dermatitis) and/ or brown staining (hyper-pigmentation) Depth: usually shallow Wound margins: irregular Exudate: moderate to heavy Edema: pitting or nonpitting; possible induration and cellulitis Skin temp: normal; warm to touch Granulation: frequently present Infection: less common	Color: base of wound, pale/ pallor on elevation; dependent rubor Skin: shiny, taut, thin, dry, hair loss on lower extremities, atrophy of subcutaneous tissue Depth: deep Wound margins: even Exudate: minimal Edema: variable Skin temp: decreased/cold Granulation tissue: rarely present Infection: frequent (signs may be subtle) Necrosis, eschar, gangrene may be present	Color: normal skin tones; trophic skin changes, fissuring and/or callus formation Depth: variable Wound margins: well defined Exudate: variable Edema: cellulitis, erythema, and induration common Skin temp: warm Granulation tissue: frequently present Infection: frequent Necrotic tissue variable, gangrene uncommon Reflexes usually diminished Altered gait; orthopaedic deformities common

	Venous Insufficiency (Stasis)	Arterial Insufficiency	Peripheral Neuropathy
Perfusion	Pain • Minimal unless infected or desiccated Peripheral pulses • Present/palpable Capillary refill • Normal—less than 3 seconds	Pain • Intermittent claudication • Resting • Positional • Nocturnal Peripheral pulses • Absent or diminished Capillary refill • Delayed—more than 3 seconds • ABI $<$ 0.8	Pain • Diminished sensitivity to touch • Reduced response to pin prick, usually painless Peripheral pulses • Palpable/present Capillary refill • Normal

	Measures to improve venous return
	• Surgical obliteration of damaged veins
	• Elevation of legs
	• Compression therapy to provide at least 30 mm Hg compression at ankle, using
	• Short stretch bandages (e.g., Setopress, Surepress, Comprilan)
	• Therapeutic support stockings
	  • Unna boot
	  • Profore 4-layer wrap
	  • Compression pumps
	Topical therapy
	• Goals: absorb exudate, maintain moist wound surface (e.g., alginate, foam, hydrocolloid dressings)
		Measures to improve tissue perfusion
		• Revascularization if possible
		• Medications to improve red blood cell transit through narrowed vessels
		• Lifestyle changes (no tobacco, no caffeine, no constrictive garments, avoidance of cold)
		• Hydration
		• Measures to prevent trauma to tissues (appropriate foot-wear at all times)
		Topical therapy
		• Dry uninfected necrotic wound; keep dry
		• Dry infected wound, immediate referral for surgical debridement/ aggressive antibiotic therapy
		• Open wound
		  • Moist wound healing
		  • Nonocclusive dressings (e.g., solid hydrogels) or cautious use of occlusive dressings
		  • Aggressive treatment of any infection
			Measures to eliminate trauma
			• Pressure relief for heel ulcers
			• "Offloading" for plantar ulcers (bedfast or contact casting or orthopaedic shoes)
			• Appropriate footwear
			Tight glucose control
			Aggressive infection control (debridement of any necrotic tissue, orthopaedic consult for exposed bone, antibiotic coverage)
			Topical therapy
			• Cautious use of occlusive dressings
			• Dressings to absorb exudate/keep surface moist

Algorithm to Determine Wound Etiology

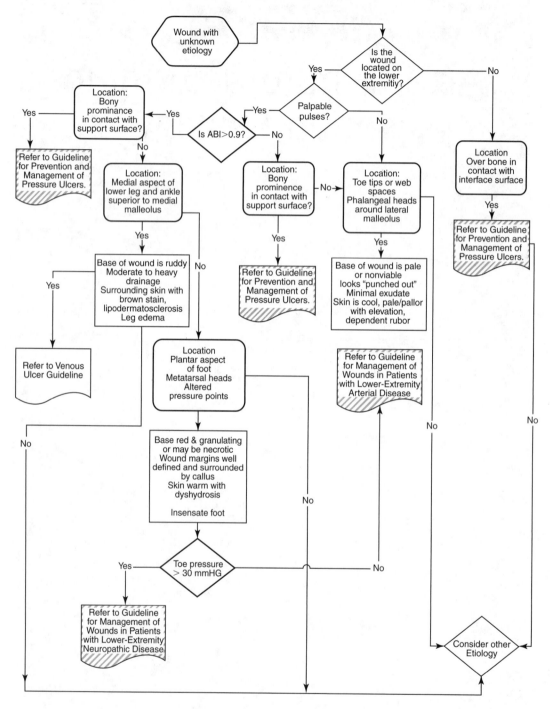

Source: From *Guideline for the Management of Wounds in Patients with Lower-Extremity Arterial Disease.* Copyright 2002 by the Wound, Ostomy, Continence Nurses Society.

INDEX